FETAL LIVER TRANSPLANTATION

DEVELOPMENTS IN HEMATOLOGY AND IMMUNOLOGY

Lijnen, H.R., Collen, D. and Verstraete, M., eds: Synthetic Substrates in Clinical Blood Coagulation Assays. 1980. ISBN 90-247-2409-0

Smit Sibinga, C.Th., Das, P.C. and Forfar, J.O., eds: Paediatrics and Blood Transfusion. 1982. ISBN 90-247-2619-0

Fabris, N., ed: Immunology and Ageing. 1982. ISBN 90-247-2640-9

Hornstra, G.: Dietary Fats, Prostanoids and Arterial Thrombosis. 1982. ISBN 90-247-2667-0

Smit Sibinga, C.Th., Das, P.C. and Loghem, van J.J., eds: Blood Transfusion and Problems of Bleeding. 1982. ISBN 90-247-3058-9

Dormandy, J., ed: Red Cell Deformability and Filterability. 1983. ISBN 0-89838-578-4

Smit Sibinga, C.Th., Das, P.C. and Taswell, H.F., eds: Quality Assurance in Blood Banking and Its Clinical Impact. 1984. ISBN 0-89838-618-7

Besselaar, A.M.H.P. van den, Gralnick, H.R. and Lewis, S.M., eds: Thromboplastin Calibration and Oral Anticoagulant Control. 1984. ISBN 0-89838-637-3

Fondu, P. and Thijs, O., eds: Haemostatic Failure in Liver Disease. 1984. ISBN 0-89838-640-3

Smit Sibinga, C.Th., Das, P.C. and Opelz, G., eds: Transplantation and Blood Transfusion. 1984. ISBN 0-89838-686-1

Schmid-Schönbein, H., Wurzinger, L.J. and Zimmerman, R.E., eds: Enzyme Activation in Blood-Perfused Artificial Organs. 1985. ISBN 0-89838-704-3

Dormandy, J., ed: Blood Filtration and Blood Cell Deformability. 1985. ISBN 0-89838-714-0

Smit Sibinga, C.Th., Das, P.C. and Seidl, S., eds: Plasma Fractionation and Blood Transfusion. 1985. ISBN 0-89838-761-2

Dawids, S. and Bantjes, A., eds: Blood Compatible Materials and their Testing. 1986. ISBN 0-89838-813-9

Smit Sibinga, C.Th., Das, P.C. and Greenwalt, T.J., eds: Future Developments in Blood Banking. 1986. ISBN 0-89838-824-4

Berlin, A., Dean, J., Draper, M.H., Smith, E.M.B. and Spreafico, F., eds: Immunotoxicology. 1987. ISBN 0-89838-843-0

Ottenhoff, T. and De Vries, R.: Recognition of *M. leprae* antigens. 1987. ISBN 0-89838-887-2

Touraine, J.-L., Gale, R.P. and Kochupillai, V., eds: Fetal Liver Transplantation. 1987. ISBN 0-89838-975-5

Fetal liver transplantation

Reprinted from Thymus, International Journal of Thymology, Immunobiology, and Clinical Immunology, Volume 10, Number 1−2 (1987)

edited by

JEAN-LOUIS TOURAINE

Hôpital Edouard Herriot, Lyon, France

ROBERT PETER GALE

Transplantation Biology Program, University of California, Los Angeles, U.S.A.

VINOD KOCHUPILLAI

Institute Rotary, Cancer Hospital, New Delhi, India

1987 **MARTINUS NIJHOFF PUBLISHERS**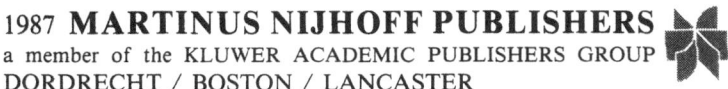
a member of the KLUWER ACADEMIC PUBLISHERS GROUP
DORDRECHT / BOSTON / LANCASTER

Distributors

for the United States and Canada: Kluwer Academic Publishers, P.O. Box 358, Accord Station, Hingham, MA 02018-0358, USA
for the UK and Ireland: Kluwer Academic Publishers, MTP Press Limited, Falcon House, Queen Square, Lancaster LA1 1RN, UK
for all other countries: Kluwer Academic Publishers Group, Distribution Center, P.O. Box 322, 3300 AH Dordrecht, The Netherlands

Library of Congress Cataloging in Publication Data

Fetal liver transplantation.

  (Developments in hematology and immunology)
  "Reprinted from Thymus, international journal of
thymology, immunobiology, and clinical immunology,
volume 10, number 1-2 (1987)."
    1. Fetal liver cells--Transplantation. 2. Aplastic
anemia--Treatment. 3. Leukemia--Treatment.
I. Touraine, J. L. (Jean Louis) II. Gale, Robert
Peter. III. Kochupillai, Vinod. IV. Thymus. V. Series.
[DNLM: 1. Anemia, Aplastic--therapy. 2. Bone Marrow--
transplantation. 3. Fetus--surgery. 4. Hematopoietic
Stem Cells. 5. Leukemia, Myelocytic--therapy.
6. Liver--transplantation. W1 DE997VZK / WI 700 F419]
RD546.F47 1987   616.1'52   87-24059
ISBN-13: 978-94-010-8011-8   e-ISBN-13: 978-94-009-3365-1
DOI: 10.1007/978-94-009-3365-1

Copyright

CONTENTS

Synopsis and prospectives on fetal liver transplantation
R.P. Gale, J.-L. Touraine & V. Kochupillai — 1

Survey of experimental data on fetal liver transplantation
C. Royo, J.-L. Touraine, P. Veyron & A. Aitouche — 5

Sustained recovery of hematopoiesis and immunity following transplantation of fetal liver cells in dogs
R.E. Champling, G. Cain, K. Stitzel & R.P. Gale — 13

Variation of treatment conditions alter the outcome of fetal liver transplantation in dogs
O. Prümmer, W. Calvo & T.M. Fliedner — 19

What kind of morphologically recognizable haemopoietic cells do we inject when doing foetal liver infusion in man?
E. Kelemen, M. Jánossa, W. Calvo, T.M. Fliedner, M. Bofill & G. Janossy — 33

Development of the immune system in human fetal liver
R.P. Gale — 45

Ontogeny of T lymphocyte differentiation in the human fetus: Acquisition of phenotype and functions
C. Royo, J.-L. Touraine & O. de Bouteiller — 57

Fetal tissue transplantation, bone marrow transplantation and prospective gene therapy in severe immunodeficiencies and enzyme deficiencies
J.-L. Touraine, M.G. Roncarolo, C. Royo & F. Touraine — 75

Fetal liver transplantation in aplastic anemia and leukemia
R.P. Gale — 89

Fetal liver infusion in aplastic anaemia
V. Kochupillai, S. Sharma, S. Francis, A. Nanu, S. Mathew, P. Bhatia, H. Dua, L. Kumar, S. Aggarwal, S. Singh, S. Kumar, A. Karak & M. Bhargava — 95

Bone marrow recovery following fetal liver infusion (FLI) in aplastic anaemia: Morphological studies
M. Bhargava, A.K. Karak, S. Sharma & V. Kochupillai — 103

Advances in experimental studies and clinical application of fetal liver cells
Chu Tse Wu & Gen Yad Ye — 109

Fetal liver infusion in acute myelogenous leukaemia
V. Kochupillai, S. Sharma, S. Francis, A. Nanu, I.C. Verma, H. Dua, L. Kumar, S. Aggarwal & S. Singh 117

Studies on engraftment following fetal liver infusion
P. Bhatia, V. Kochupillai, S. Mathew, N.K. Mehra, A. Nanu, N. Jayasuryan, S. Sharma, S. Francis & P.S.N. Menon 125

HLA status following fetal liver transplantation in aplastic anaemia and acute myeloid leukaemia
N.K. Mehra, V. Taneja, B. Jhinghon, T. Chaudhuri, S. Sharma & V. Kochupillai 131

Marrow uptake index (MUI): A quantitative scintigraphic study of bone marrow in aplastic anaemia
A.K. Padhy, A. Garg, V. Kochupillai, P.G. Gopinath & A.K. Basu 137

A comparison between ALG and bone marrow transplantation in treatment of severe aplastic anemia
B. Speck, A. Gratwohl, C. Nissen, B. Osterwalder, A. Würsch, A. Tichelli, A. Lori, P. Reusser, M. Jeannet & E. Signer 147

Thymus 10:1–4 (1987)
© Martinus Nijhoff Publishers, Dordrecht

Synopsis and prospectives on fetal liver transplantation

ROBERT PETER GALE, JEAN-LOUIS TOURAINE[1] and VINOD KOCHUPILLAI

Los Angeles, USA; Lyon, France; and New-Delhi, India

(*Accepted 19th May 1987*)

Summary. Over 300 individuals have received fetal liver transplants for a spectrum of disorders including immunodeficiencies, aplastic anemia, leukemia and genetic disorders. In some instances, the objective has been to reconstitute the immune system from fetal liver-derived lymphoid stem cells. In aplastic anemia and leukemia two distinct approaches have been used: engraftment of fetal liver-derived hematopoietic stem cells or attempts to stimulate recovery of autologous hematopoiesis via factors produced by fetal liver. In genetic disorders, partial engraftment of fetal liver-derived hematopoietic and hepatic cells has been investigated. This report critically reviews data presented at a symposium on fetal liver transplantation in New-Delhi, 1–5 February 1986.

On 1–5 February, 1986, a symposium on fetal liver transplantation was held at the All India Institute for Medical Sciences in New Delhi. This issue contains presentations from this meeting. Additionally there were two discussion sessions involving most of the participants. In this manuscript, we review conclusions of these discussions and consider future directions of fetal liver transplantation in man.

Fetal liver transplantation has been attempted in four major types of disorders: immune deficiency, aplastic anemia, leukemia and genetic or metabolic disorders. In so far as these disorders are diverse, the objectives of fetal liver transplantation will typically vary.

In immune deficiency disorders, the usual objective of fetal liver transplantation is to reconstitute the immune system from fetal liver derived lymphoid stem cells. Considerable data were presented indicating that in all species studied, including man, fetal liver contains both T- and B-lymphoid progenitors cells.

Patients with severe combined immunodeficiency (SCID) lack a functional immune system, and it is therefore not necessary to administer pre-transplant immune suppression to achieve engraftment, in most instances. Fetal liver transplants are typically carried out in individuals who

---

[1] *Address for offprints*: Dr. J.-L. Touraine, Hôpital Edouard Herriot, 5 place d'Arsonval, F-69437 Lyon Cedex 8, France.

lack an HLA-identical donor for bone marrow transplantation. Some of these transplants have involved transfer of only fetal liver cells whereas, in other instances, both fetal liver and fetal thymus have been given. The usefulness of the associated fetal thymus, suggested by several animal experiments, has not yet been conclusively established as significantly beneficial in man since few comparative data on fetal liver transplants with or without thymus are available.

Sustained engraftment with reconstitution of immune function has been achieved in a number of patients. Full immunological reconstitution has, in particular, involved normal T-cell functions, without any restriction, despite the complete HLA mismatch between donor stem cells (and their T-cell progeny) on the one hand, and host cells on the other hand. The optimal age of fetal livers, for transplantation in infants with SCID, is suggested to be 8–13 weeks post-fecundation, for transplantation in infants with SCID, and certainly fetuses greater than 20 weeks may be associated with an increased risk of causing graft-versus-host disease (GvHD). The likelihood of GvHD may also be increased when thymocytes from fetuses at a late stage of development are transplanted along with fetal liver cells. Frequently several different fetal liver transplants had to be performed some weeks apart before cells from one fetal liver successfully engraft. Immune reconstitution may be complete or may involve only T-cells. Failure of B-cell engraftment is likely related to residual B-cells in the recipient. These host B-cells become able to differentiate into immunoglobulin-secreting plasma cells following development of T-cells, despite their different HLA phenotype.

Patients with incomplete immunodeficiency could also be treated by fetal liver transplantation, but may require pre-transplant immune suppression, as performed before bone marrow transplantation in such cases. The relative efficacy of fetal liver versus HLA-haplo-identical, T-cell-depleted bone marrow transplantation has not been resolved, but the lower complication rate of fetal liver transplantation has been established.

Two approaches have been used in fetal liver transplantation for aplastic anemia. One approach is to try to achieve sustained engraftment of fetal liver-derived hematopoietic stem cells similar to bone marrow transplantation. Sustained engraftment has not yet been demonstrated following fetal liver transplants in patients with aplastic anemia, but none of these studies has used the level of pre-transplant immune suppression which is anticipated to be required based on studies in dogs. Presently, it seems premature to attempt these studies in man until additional data are available in pre-clinical models.

A second approach in aplastic anemia is to infuse fetal liver cells in an attempt to stimulate recovery of autologous hematopoiesis. Two studies presented data suggesting a beneficial effect of fetal liver infusions in this regard. Another study claimed a benefit of infusion of a cell-free sonicate of fetal liver cells. Experimental data in mice also suggested an effect on immune and hematologic function, mediated via factors derived from fetal liver cells.

The concept that fetal liver cells or factors derived from them might stimulate autologous hematopoiesis was discussed extensively. Two investigators felt that there were reasonably convincing data in man. Others felt that the heterogeneity of this disease and its possible outcomes made randomized, double-blind trials essential. The consensus was to attempt to perform these trials in the new future. It is also likely worthwhile to initiate more detailed studies of putative, biologically active factors, present in fetal liver and potentially able to stimulate hematopoiesis.

In leukemia, both fetal liver transplantation and fetal liver infusion have been attempted. Sustained engraftment was reported in two patients receiving pre-transplant chemotherapy and radiation, but not in most individuals. As in aplastic anemia, doses of drugs and radiation in most studies would not have been expected to be adequate to achieve sustained engraftment, based on studies in dogs. Additional data derived from studies of HLA-partially matched, T-cell-depleted bone marrow transplants also suggest that these conditioning regimens are not sufficiently intensive to ensure sustained engraftment. Thus, presently there are no convincing data regarding fetal liver transplantation in leukemia and additional results from pre-clinical models are needed. These data in experimental animals will probably be provided shortly; clinical trials will then be able to evaluate fetal liver transplantation in patients with advanced leukemia.

Fetal liver infusions, without attempts at engraftment, have also been evaluated in leukemia. Two approaches have been used: infusions to expedite recovery following induction chemotherapy (similar to aplastic anemia) and infusions given while in remission to prolong remission duration. It is also possible, albeit unlikely, that fetal liver cells might temporarily engraft under these conditions.

Data supporting a role for fetal liver infusions in leukemia were not absolutely convincing. The primary determinant of the rate of recovery following induction chemotherapy is the efficacy of leukemia eradication. This efficacy is already highly variable in patients receiving chemotherapy without additional measures and it would be difficult to detect an effect of fetal liver infusion, even if present, in a limited number of patients. It is also very uncertain whether or not fetal liver infusion during remission would extend remission duration, for several reasons. Trials of immunotherapy for human leukemias have been mostly unsuccessful to date. Furthermore, the beneficial anti-leukemia effect associated with allogeneic bone marrow transplantation, termed graft-versus-leukemia (GvL), typically occurs in the context of GvHD, a reaction less likely to develop at a significant degree following fetal liver transplantation.

Fetal liver transplants have been used to treat genetic and metabolic disorders. Two individuals have received transplants for thalassemia. Both were reported to benefit transiently but data supporting this conclusion were not presented. The intensity of pre-transplant conditioning in these individuals was probably insufficient to achieve sustained engraftment. Whether factors derived from fetal liver might increase hemoglobin F synthesis is unknown.

Attempts to correct genetic disorders such as Fabry disease, Gaucher disease or Niemann-Pick disease by temporary engraftment of fetal liver-derived heptocytes and hematopoietic cells were also reported. In these individuals, the fetal liver cells were given repeatedly, at 6–12 month intervals, intraperitoneally. Patients received azathioprine and corticosteroids to enhance the temporary persistence of the fetal hepatic cells. One of us reported beneficial results in these patients, particularly those without nervous system involvement. Evidence of persistence of these cells was indirect, based on elevated levels of α-fetoprotein, on decreased levels of substrates, and on maintained clinical improvement. The treatment of metabolic disorders by this approach is still investigational and, due to the diversity of diseases, a precise evaluation of the degree of effectiveness in each condition will probably require a few additional years. This mode of treatment will also prepare the gene therapies that will probably develop in the near future for certain of these diseases.

In conclusion, trials of fetal liver transplantation or infusion are advancing. Success is now frequent in patients with SCID who can be definitively cured by this procedure. In hematological disorders there is a need for controlled trials to prove whether fetal liver infusion is efficacious. Data in dogs clearly indicate that it is possible to successfully transplant a single fully DLA-mismatched fetal liver following appropriate conditioning. As soon as technical details evolve, it should be possible to evaluate this approach in patients with advanced leukemia and possibly those with severe aplastic anemia. In vitro studies of factors derived from fetal liver that stimulate hematopoiesis may also prove interesting.

The next conference to discuss these data was tentatively scheduled to be at the Claude Bernard University in Lyon, France.

Thymus 10:5–12 (1987)

Survey of experimental data on fetal liver transplantation

C. ROYO,[1] J.-L. TOURAINE, P. VEYRON and A. AITOUCHE

Transplantation and Immunobiology Unit, Pavillon P, Hôpital Edouard Herriot, F-69437 Lyon Cédex 08, France

(*Accepted 19 May 1987*)

Key words: Animal models, fetal liver, fetal thymus, transplantation, bone marrow, hematopoietic stem cells

Summary. Fetal liver transplantation has been shown to induce hematogological and immunological reconstitution in irradiated rodents, dogs, horses and sheep. Engraftment and reconstitution without GvHD has been readily obtained using histocompatible donors. When mismatched fetal donors were used, a comparatively larger number of donor cells was required, in addition to pre-treatment of host with higher doses of irradiation or irradiation plus chemotherapy. Stem cell suspensions devoid of any T lymphocyte can be transplanted across major histocompatibility barrier without inducing overt GvHD. The transplanted animals become tolerant to both donor and host grafts.

Introduction

Severe congenital immune disorders and inherited or acquired hematological diseases can be cured by bone marrow transplantation (BMT)[20, 21, 15, 22]. However when no HLA-identical donor is available, BMT is responsible for severe graft-versus-host disease (GvHD). Since GvHD is induced by the T lymphocytes present in the transplant and which react with host tissues [8, 10], BMT from non-HLA-genotypically identical donor must be preceded by T-cell depletion of the bone marrow. This manoeuvre does reduce the incidence of GvHD but it is associated with an increased risk of take failure, EBV-induced lymphomas or incomplete reconstitution [22]. It is therefore of great interest that fetal liver stem cells can reconstitute the hematopoietic and lymphopoietic systems of both animals and humans without severe GvHD, even in cases of full donor-host incompatibility [22–24, 13]. Since the pioneering work of Uphoff [24] in 1958, much has been learned in the fields of experimental and clinical fetal liver transplantation (FLT). Much still remains to be discovered for the optimal use of this mode of treatment in all varieties of severe hematological and immunological diseases.

---

[1]Author for correspondence.

The purpose of this paper is to review briefly the experimental data on FLT and to indicate the questions remaining unsolved. Most experimental studies have been carried out in mice and occasionally in rats [6, 3, 13, 9, 18]; a few other analyses, however, have been performed in larger and outbred animals: dogs [17, 5], horses [16], sheep [25, 4] and mini-pigs [1].

Experimental FLT in mice

The mouse has been extensively used as an animal model for experimental FLT following irradiation [6, 3, 13, 9, 18].

Main characteristics of mouse fetal liver cells

The comparison of mouse fetal liver cells and adult bone marrow cells has shown a much lower number of immunocompetent lymphocytes and a higher ratio of erythroid to granuloid cells in the former than in the latter: 8.3 in fetal liver versus 0.7 in bone marrow [13]. There is virtually no differentiated T lymphocytes in the fetal liver, especially until day 16, i.e. 5 days prior to birth. However, stem cells and precursor cells for all hematopoietic and lymphopoietic cell lines have been conclusively demonstrated in the fetal liver. The frequency of prothymocytes has been found to be significantly lower in the fetal liver than in the adult bone marrow (10 times less when an equal number of nucleated cells from both tissues was compared) in 12–16 day-old fetuses [2]. The frequency of colony-forming-unit-spleen (CFU-s) was also lower in the fetal liver than in the adult bone marrow, when measured in comparative conditions, but the difference was of a smaller order of magnitude: 4 times less in fetal liver than in bone marrow [2, 13]. The absence of T lymphocytes and the lower number of prothymocytes explain the lack of GvHD and the slight delay in T-cell reconstitution following FLT as compared with BMT. Whether or not this low frequency of cells of the T-lineage is responsible for some reduction of takeability or of hematopoietic development following transplantation is still a matter for further investigation. The role of cells of this lineage is suggested by the reduced take of T-cell-depleted bone marrow transplants, but the mechanism is still speculative.

The proliferative capacities of fetal liver stem cells appeared to be higher than those of bone marrow stem cells, as indicated by the more rapid increase of fetal liver-derived CFU than bone marrow-derived CFU in the spleen following transplantation [13, 19]. In vitro studies of fetal liver cells between day 12 and birth have not led to definitive conclusions regarding the optimal age for FLT. Most studies have been performed using cells of 14 to 18 days post-fecundation.

Syngeneic FLT

Reconstitution of irradiated syngeneic mice can be obtained with very low numbers of CFU-s from the fetal liver: transplantation of 30 fetal liver-

Table 1. Survival of lethally irradiated mice following syngeneic FLT or BMT.

Number of transplanted cells	Survival at day 30
30 fetal liver-derived CFU-s (18 days) (i.e. 0.5–0.7×10^6 nucleated cells)	50%
30 adult bone marrow-derived CFU-s (i.e. 0.1×10^6 nucleated cells)	0%
120 fetal liver-derived CFU-s (18 days) (i.e. 2–3×10^6 nucleated cells)	80%
120 adult bone marrow-derived CFU-s (i.e. 0.8–1.0×10^6 nucleated cells)	80%

From B. Löwenberg (ref. 13).

derived CFU-s enabled 50% of the animals to survive whereas none of the mice transplanted with the same number of adult bone marrow-derived CFU-s survived [13]. When a larger number of CFU-s were transplanted, a larger proportion of mice recovered from the radiation effects and it was calculated that 120 fetal liver-derived CFU-s or 240 bone marrow-derived CFU-s were required for an 80% survival (Table 1). Due to the lower proportion of CFU-s among nucleated cells of the fetal liver than the bone marrow, the number of nucleated cells injected to obtain these quantities of CFU-s were 2–3×10^6 from the fetal liver and 0.8 1.0×10^6 from the bone marrow.

The hematopoietic reconstitution started 5 days following the intravenous administration of fetal liver cells and proceeded until day 13 [13]. Lymphocytes, granulocytes and reticulocytes normalized between days 15 and 25 and trombocytes at day 30. The rapidity of reconstitution depends on the number of injected cells. In addition, we have observed an influence of the route of administration, reconstitution being slightly delayed following intraperitoneal injection of the cells as compared with intravenous administration. A slightly increased number of fetal liver cells also appears to be required for the use by the intraperitoneal route to achieve the same degree of survival and full reconstitution as following intravenous FLT. To evaluate immunological reconstitution, B. Löwenberg analyzed in vitro mitogen responsiveness of spleen cells to Concanavalin A and to lipopolysaccharide [13]. He found a subnormal proliferative response at one month and a normal response at two months, suggesting that the proliferative capacities of T and B lymphocytes require between 13 and 16 days following FLT. R. Fleischman et al. [7] and B. Mintz [14] have shown that totipotent hematopoietic stem cells from the fetal liver could induce reconstitution of erythroid cells in genetically anemic fetuses when injected via the placental circulation. In these conditions of intrafetal transplantation of fetal liver cells, and using computerized statistical models, the authors have shown that some animals must have been seeded by only a single donor cell and that this single stem cell has been sufficient for reconstitution.

Table 2. Survival of lethally irradiated mice following allogeneic FLT or BMT (CBA→C57B1/6).

Number of transplanted cells	Survival at day 30	Survival at day 100
1200 fetal liver-derived CFU-s (18 days) (i.e. 20–30 × 10^6 nucleated cells)	88%	39%
1200 adult bone marrow-derived CFU-s (i.e. 4–5 × 10^6 nucleated cells)	80%	2%

From B. Löwenberg (Ref. 13).

Allogeneic FLT

To provide survival of irradiated mice, a larger number of cells was required from allogeneic donors than from syngeneic donors. In the C57B1/6-CBA combination, at least 80% of mice survived over 30 days following transplantation of either 1200 fetal liver-derived CFU-s or 1200 adult bone marrow-derived CFU-s [13]. At day 100, however, the percentage of surviving mice was significantly reduced (Table 2): 39% following FLT, probably due to insufficient reconstitution, and 2% only following BMT, due to GvHD [13]. This allogeneic repression, which is responsible for poorer long-term results of allogeneic FLT than syngeneic FLT, may be related in some way to the hybrid resistance [11]. It could be overcome by increasing the number of fetal liver cells or by the addition of thymocytes syngeneic with the fetal liver cells. In the CBA-Balb/c combination, we have observed that 5 × 10^6 fetal liver cells administered intraperitoneally were not sufficient whereas 20 × 10^6 or more fetal liver cells induced a 70% survival at 3 months, with hematological and immunological reconstitution. The beneficial effect of the addition of fetal thymocytes to FLT has been initially reported by M. Bortin et al. [3] and confirmed by B. Löwenberg et al. [13]. Increase take of FLT, accelerated reconstitution and inhibition of GvHD have been reported by these authors to result from this addition of fetal thymocytes. This effect was only observed when fetal thymocytes were syngeneic to fetal liver cells. No benefit of fetal thymocytes was noticed when FLT was performed in a syngeneic host [12]. Adult thymocytes were detrimental since they induced GvHD.

Allogeneic FLT can result in a high rate of survival of lethally irradiated mice, provided that an adequate number of cells is transplanted. By contrast with allogeneic bone marrow transplantation across major H2 barrier, FLT is not associated with severe acute GvHD. In some strain combinations, delayed mortality has been observed, as a consequence of insufficient reconstitution or of delayed GvHD. Such a delayed GvHD was unfrequent when donor age was 14 days; it could be seen with ages of 16–18 days. Using 14 day-old fetuses as donor (a condition which frequently required several donors for a single recipient mouse in order to

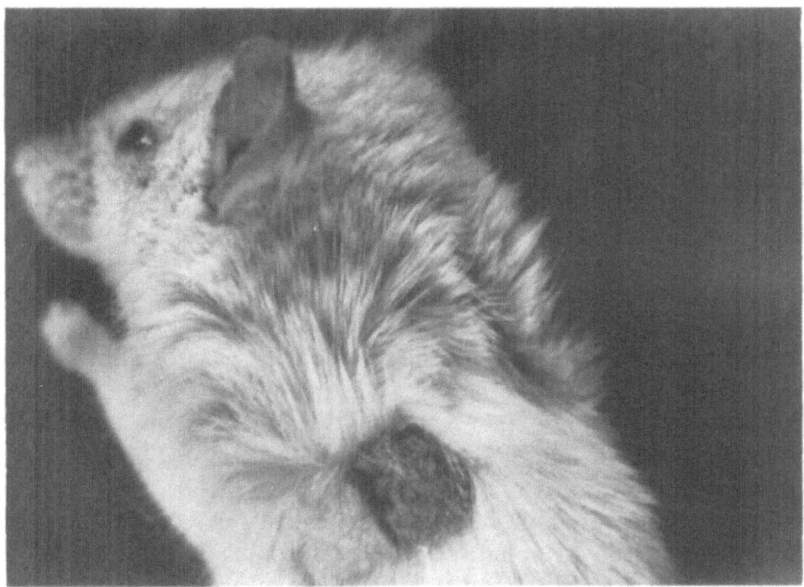

Figure 1. CBA mouse (H2-k) transplanted with fetal liver cells from Balb/c strain (H2-d). This mouse is now tolerant both to donor and host tissues and does not reject syngeneic (CBA, top) as well as allogeneic (Balb/c, bottom) skin transplants. This mouse would, however, reject a third party skin transplant.

transplant a sufficient number of cells), full hematological and immuno-logical reconstitution could be obtained from donor cells in less than 2 months. The recipient mouse frequently developed a transient and moderate enlargement of the spleen, as compared with syngeneic controls, but no overt GvHD occurred, either acutely or chronically. These results suggest that H2-mismatched stem cells do not induce GvHD after they have matured into T lymphocytes in the allogeneic host. The delayed GvHD occasionally observed after 16–18 day-old FLT possibly result from the few cells already engaged in T-cell differentiation and which are present in the liver at the end of the mouse fetal development.

Following allogeneic FLT, mice demonstrated immunological tolerance both to donor and to host tissues. CBA mice transplanted with Balb/c fetal livers did not reject skin transplants from Balb/c as well as from CBA mice (Figure 1). They rejected, however, a third party skin transplant, e.g. C57Bl/6 skin in 13 days. Control mice rejected these allogeneic transplants in 11–12 days. From these data, it can be concluded that the immunodeficiency remaining 3 months after irradiation and allogeneic FLT is extremely mild but that a specific tolerance to donor antigens is present. This tolerance is stable and can be demonstrated after more than one year. In these mice, we have shown that virtually all T lymphocytes are of donor H2-type.

In additional experiments using cryopreserved fetal liver cells from 14 day-old mouse fetuses, we have seen a 50% loss of viable cells but a preserved capacity to reconstitute irradiated allogeneic mice. Cryopreservation with the presently available techniques can therefore be used for FLT experiments provided that cell procurement is calculated to be initially twice as large as when fresh cells are transplanted.

FLT in dogs

Syngeneic and allogeneic FLT have been shown to be able to restore hematopoiesis and lymphopoiesis in lethally irradiated dogs [5, 17]. Fetal livers were obtained from 50–53 day-old fetuses, i.e. 10 days before the expected birth. Fetal liver cells were sometimes cryopreserved. They were able to rapidly engraft and induce reconstitution in histocompatible siblings exposed to total body irradiation (14–18 Gys). The various cell lines were demonstrated to develop in peripheral blood from the second week after transplantation. A faster B-cell than T-cell recovery was observed. The proliferative response of peripheral blood lymphocytes to phytomitogens was normal at 3 months. The rapidity of granulocyte and platelet recovery was related to the number of CFU-GM transfused. Proliferating bone marrow cells were of donor origin, as shown by chromosomal analyses when donors and recipients were of opposite sex. A few host lymphocytes, however, persisted in the initial phase of recovery. No severe GvHD was subsequently observed [17]. Allogeneic FLT required high dose total body irradiation (18 Gys) or 16 Gys total body irradiation plus methothrexate or cyclosporin. When a more moderate conditioning was used, no engraftment of mismatched FLT was obtained [5]. Mild GvHD, especially of the delayed type, or auto-immune manifestations were occasionally observed and may suggest either to use slightly younger fetuses or a mild immunosuppressive therapy for some weeks following FLT. Experiments in dogs have shown that, although the technique may still be improved, FLT from a single donor can reconstitute hematopoiesis and lymphopoiesis in DLA-mismatched animals.

FLT in horses

Horses with combined immunodeficiency have been treated with FLT by Perryman et al. [16]. Donor ages ranged from 68 days to 110 days postfecundation. Two out of nine horses had a sustained engraftment following transplantation of both fetal liver and fetal thymus. They survived respectively for 8 and more than 11 months following FLT. One of these 2 horses died with GvHD manifestations of the chronic type. The occurrence and severity of GvHD in 4 of the 9 animals appeared to be related to the age of the fetal donor and to the presence of numerous fetal thymocytes.

FLT in sheep

FLT has resulted in reconstitution of 7 out of 40 sheep conditioned by lethal irradiation [4]. No overt GvHD was seen. In other experiments, the association of fetal bone marrow cells to fetal liver cells seemed to be beneficial for engraftment [25].

Conclusion

FLT has been shown to be able to induce reconstitution of lethally irradiated animals from various species. Engraftment of allogeneic stem cells from the fetal liver appears to be somewhat more difficult and requiring a larger number of cells than when using perfectly matched donors. However, unlike allogeneic BMT, GvHD was unfrequent, especially when fetal donors were relatively young. If simplistic rules had to be formulated in deduction from these experimental data, they could be summarized as follows:

— the intravenous route needs relatively less cells than the intraperitoneal route;

— the more histoincompatible the donor, the larger the number of donor cells and the more potent the immune suppression of the host;

— the more immature the fetal donor, the lower the incidence of GvHD but also the more difficult the engraftment;

— fetal livers obtained at the end of gestation provide more cells and are associated with a relatively higher rate of engraftment, but also with more GvHD. The choice may thus be between early fetal livers from several donors and late fetal liver from a single donor; GvHD is more frequent in the latter condition, difficulty in take of mismatched stem cells is perhaps slightly higher in the former.

References

1. Andreani M, De Biagi M, Centis F, Manna M, Agostinelli F, Filipetti A, Gaudenzi G, Muretto P, Grianti C, Sotti G, Rigon A, Lucarelli G (1985) Fetal liver transplantation in the mini-pig. In: Gale RP, Touraine JL, Lucarelli G (eds) Progress in Clinical and Biological Research: Fetal liver transplantation. New York: Alan R. Liss, Inc., p. 205.
2. Boersma WJA (1983) Prothymocytes in mouse fetal liver. Thymus 5:419.
3. Bortin MM, Saltzstein EC (1969) Graft-versus-host inhibition: Fetal liver and thymus cells to minimize secondary disease. Science 164:316.
4. Bunch C, Wood WG, Kelly SJ (1985) Fetal hemopoietic-cell transplantation in sheep: An approach to the cellular control of hemoglobin switching. In Gale RP, Touraine JL, Lucarelli G (eds) Progress in Clinical and Biological Research: Fetal Liver Transplantation. New York: Alan R. Liss Inc., p. 219.
5. Champlin RE, Cain G, Stitzel KA, Gale RP (1987) Sustained recovery of hematopoiesis and immunity following transplantation of fetal liver cells in dogs. Thymus, this issue.

6. Crouch BG (1959) Transplantation of fetal hemopoietic tissues into irradiated mice and rats. In: Proc. Seventh Congress of the Eur. Soc. for Haematology, London, p. 973.
7. Fleischman RA, Cluster RP, Mintz B (1982) Totipotent hematopoietic stem cells: Normal self-renewal and differentiation after transplantation between mouse fetuses: Cell 30:351.
8. Grebe SC, Streilen JW (1976) Graft-versus-host reactions: A review. Adv. Immunol. 22:119.
9. Kelemen E, Gulya E, Szabo (Hatvan)(1980) Xenogeneic transfer of fetal liver- and adult bone marrow-derived hemopoietic cells in rodents. In: Lucarelli G, Fliedern TM, Gale RP (eds) Fetal liver transplantation. Amsterdam: Excerpta Medica, p. 168.
10. Korngold R, Sprent J (1982) Features of T-cells causing H-2 restricted lethal graft-versus-host disease across minor histocompatibility barrier. J. Exp. Med. 155:182.
11. Goodman JW, Wheeler HB (1968) Factors that modify poor growth of parental marrow cells in F1 hybrid mice. In: Dausset J, Hamburger J, Mathé G (eds) Advance in Transplantation. Copenhagen: Munskgaard, p. 427.
12. Goodman JW, Shinpock SG (1968) Influence of thymus cells on erythropoiesis of parental marrow in irradiated hybrid mice. Proc. Soc. Exp. Biol. Med. 129:417.
13. Löwenberg B (1975) Fetal liver cell transplantation. Thesis. Erasmus University Rotterdam. Publication of the Radiobiological Institute of the Organization for Health Research TNO, Rijswijk (ZH), The Netherlands.
14. Mintz B (1985) Renewal and differentiation of totipotent hematopoietic stem cells of the mouse after transplantation into early fetuses. In: Gale RP, Touraine JL, Lucarelli G (eds) Progress in Clinical and Biological Research: Fetal Liver Transplantation. New York: Alan R. Liss, Inc., 193:3.
15. O'Reilly R (1983) Allogeneic bone marrow transplantation: Current status and future directions. Blood 62:941.
16. Perryman LE (1980) Use of fetal tissues for immunoreconstitution in horses with severe combined immunodeficiency. In: Lucarelli G, Fliedner TM, Gale RP (eds) Fetal Liver Transplantation, Current Concepts and Future Directions. Amsterdam, Excerpta Medica, p. 183.
17. Prümmer O, Raghavarvachar A, Werner C, Calvo W, Carbonell F, Steinbach I, Fliedner TM (1985) Fetal liver transplantation in the dog. Transplantation 39:349.
18. Rabinowich H, Umiel T, Globerson A (1983) T cell progenitors in the mouse fetal liver. Transplantation 35:40.
19. Schofield R (1970) A comparative study of the repopulating potential of grafts from various haemopoietic sources: CFU repopulation. Cell Tissue Kinet 3:119.
20. Thomas ED, Storb R, Clift RA et al (1975) Bone marrow transplantation. N. Engl. J. Med. 292:832.
21. Thomas ED, Storb R, Clift RA et al (1975) Bone marrow transplantation. N. Engl. J. Med. 292:895.
22. Touraine JL, Roncarolo MG, Royo C, Touraine F (1987) Fetal tissue transplantation, bone marrow transplantation and prospective gene therapy in severe immunodeficiencies and enzyme deficiencies: Thymus, this issue.
23. Touraine JL (1983) Bone marrow and fetal liver transplantation in immunodeficiencies and inborn errors of metabolism: Lack of significant restriction of T-cell function in long-term chimeras despite HLA-mismatch. Immunological Rev. 71:103.
24. Uphoff DE (1958) Preclusion of secondary phase of irradiation syndrome by inoculation of fetal hematopoietic tissue following lethal total-body X-irradiation. J. Natl. Cancer Inst. 20:625.
25. Zanjani ED, McGlave PB, Stamatoyannopoulos G (1980) Fetal to adult transplant in sheep: A model for study of hemoglobin switching. In: Lucarelli G, Fliedner TM, Gale RP (eds) Fetal Liver Transplantation. Current Concepts. Amsterdam: Excerpta Medica, p. 108.

Thymus 10:13–18 (1987)
© Martinus Nijhoff Publishers, Dordrecht

Sustained recovery of hematopoiesis and immunity following transplantation of fetal liver cells in dogs

R.E. CHAMPLIN, G. CAIN, K. STITZEL and R.P. GALE

Department of Medicine (Hematology/Oncology), UCLA Center for The Health Sciences, Los Angeles, CA; and The Laboratory for Energy Related Health Research, University of California-Davis, Davis, Calif., USA

Summary. We studied the ability of fetal liver cells to reconstitute hematopoiesis and immunity in lethally irradiated dogs. Engraftment and sustained lymphoid and hematopoietic recovery was achieved when the recipients received a preparative regime of high-dose total body irradiation (TBI) alone followed by transplantation of DLA-identical fetal liver. The combination of high-dose TBI and cyclosporine allowed engraftment in DLA-mismatched fetal liver transplants. Typical features of graft-versus-host disease (GvHD) did not occur although autoimmune-like syndromes (myasthenia gravis, immune thrombocytopemia) were observed in some recipients. Hematopoietic recovery was rapid and complete. Recovery of T- and B-lymphocyte function was comparatively delayed, but sufficient to prevent opportunistic infections after the initial 3 months post transplant. These data indicate that cells from a single fetal liver can reconstitute hematopoiesis and immunity in DLA-mismatched recipients and suggest that human fetal liver cell transplantation may be an effective source of stem cells for patients who lack an HLA-identical donor for bone marrow transplantation.

Introduction

Graft-versus-host disease (GvHD) is a major barrier to the transplantation of allogeneic hematopoietic cells [1]. Although the pathophysiology of GvHD is incompletely defined, it is likely mediated by immunocompetent T-lymphocytes present within the transplanted graft [2]. Approximately one half of patients develop acute GvHD following bone marrow transplantation from an HLA-identical donor and the incidence of GvHD exceeds 70% among recipients of HLA-non-identical transplants [3]. Because of this problem GvHD, bone marrow transplantation is generally restricted to patients with an HLA-identical sibling donor.

Fetal liver is a major site of hematopoiesis during mid-gestation and contains abundant hematopoietic stem cells. Unlike bone marrow, fetal liver contains few immunocompetent T-lymphocytes and has only a limited capacity to induce GvHD, thus fetal liver is an attractive alternative source of hematopoietic cells for transplantation [4].

Transplantation of fetal liver cells is capable of restoring hematopoiesis and immunity in lethally irradiated rodents. The ensuing GvHD is mild and delayed compared to that which occurs following bone marrow transplantation, even if the donor and recipient are mismatched for major histocompatibility antigens [5, 6].

Supported in part by grant CA 23175 from The National Cancer Institute, USA.

Fetal liver transplantation has been utilized in man to treat a variety of hematologic and immunologic diseases. Typically, the donor of the fetal liver cells and the recipient are completely mismatched for HLA-antigens. Unfortunately, fetal liver transplantation has been frequently unsuccessful; failure to achieve sustained engraftment and incomplete restoration of hematopoiesis and immunity are major problems [7]. To study the factors required for successful fetal liver transplants we established a model in dogs.

Methods

We utilized selective breeding of dogs that were homozygous for DLA haplotypes to produce litters of uniform DLA-types (see Figure 1)[7–9]. Recipients were prepared for transplantation with total body irradiation (TBI) administered from a Co^{60} source at a dose rate of 1–2 cGy/min and given in 2 fractions 48 hours apart. Selected recipients received either methotrexate 0.25 mg/kg on days 1, 3, 6, 11 or cyclosporine 5 mg/kg twice daily beginning from day − 10 to − 1 and continued for 3 months following transplantation. Recipients and the fetal liver donors were selected to be identical for DLA antigen haplotypes (AA → AA), haplo-identical (AA → AB or AB → AC) or completely mismatched (AB → CD). Fetal livers were collected after 50–53 days gestation by hysterotomy, and a single cell suspension was obtained by fragmenting the liver and gently compressing the tissue while irrigating with tissue culture medium. Recipients received cells collected from 1–4 fetal livers to provide approximately 10^8 cells/kg recipient body weight. The fetal liver donors were selected to be sex-mismatched with the recipient; engraftment was documented by increasing peripheral blood counts, bone marrow cellularity and cytogenetic analyses. Animals were maintained in non-sterile isolation cages, and received transfusions, oral and parenteral antibiotics, as needed. Dogs were returned to open kennel conditions after 30 days.

Results

Engraftment and hematologic recovery

Forty-three dogs received fetal liver transplants. Results are summarized in Table 1. Seven consecutive dogs, receiving 14.7 Gy TBI and transplantation of DLA-identical fetal liver, had prompt and sustained engraftment. Peripheral blood granulocytes, erythrocytes and platelets recovered to normal within 3 weeks and the bone marrow cellularity recovered to normal by 1 month.

Similarly, when DLA homozygous fetal donor cells were transplanted into DLA heterozygous recipients sharing one haplotype after 14.7 Gy

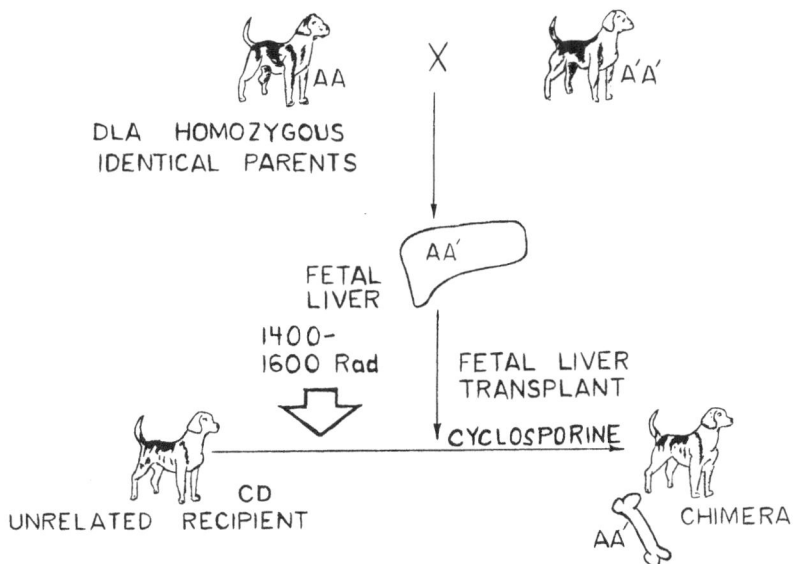

Figure 1.

TBI, 3 consecutive animals achieved sustained engraftment and hematologic recovery. Failure of engraftment occurred, however, in consecutive recipients who received 14.7 Gy TBI followed by transplantation of fetal liver cells that contained one or two DLA-haplotypes not present in the recipient (AB → AA, AC → CD).

We attempted to overcome failure of engraftment by combining 14.7 Gy TBI with post-transplant methotrexate or escalating the irradiation to 18 Gy. These regimens proved to be excessively toxic. Dogs receiving DLA haplo-identical grafts died within the first month from gastrointestinal toxicity (data not shown).

For subsequent experiments, various doses of TBI were combined with cyclosporine as preparative treatment for DLA-mismatched fetal liver transplants. 11 Gy TBI plus cyclosporine allowed initial engraftment in 4 of 9 dogs; 2 had late graft failure. This regimen had substantial toxicity, however. Six of 9 dogs receiving 14.7 Gy plus cyclosporine achieved sustained engraftment and survived over 100 days. 10 dogs received 16.1 Gy TBI plus cyclosporine. This regimen was associated with a very low rate of graft rejection with 9 of 10 dogs achieving engraftment. This regimen also had substantial toxicity; 6 dogs died from infections and/or toxicity, only 3 survived over 100 days.

Immunologic recovery

Lymphocyte recovery was variable and relatively delayed requiring 50–150 days to exceed $1.0 \times 10^9/l$. Lymphoid tissues showed partial

Table 1. Outcome of fetal liver transplants.

DLA compatibility	N	Preparative regimen (Gy)	Cyclosporine (day started)	No. with engraft.	GvHD	Survival no. > 100 days
Group 1						
compatible[a]	10	14.7	–	10	0	10
haplo-identical	4	14.7	–	0	NE[b]	0
mismatched	1	14.7	–	0	NE	0
Group 2						
mismatched	9	11.0	+(−6)	4[c]	0	1
Group 3						
haplo-identical	2	14.7	+(0)	2	0	2
mismatched	3	14.7	+(−1)	0	NE	0
mismatched	4	14.7	+(−4)	4	0	4
Group 4						
mismatched	10	16.1	+(−10)	9	0	3

[a]includes 7 DLA identical transplants and 3 receiving donor cells homozygous for DLA antigens present in the recipient (AA → AB).
[b]NE = not evaluable.
[c]2 of the 4 with engraftment subsequently exhibited late graft rejection.

restoration of B- and T-cell zones by 3 months. Response to phytohemagglutinin and reactivity in mixed lymphocyte culture recurred by 100 days; dogs were capable of rejecting cutaneous allografts by 300 days. B-cell functions evaluated by production of hemagglutinating antibody against sheep erythrocytes also recovered by 3 months. Nineteen of the 29 dogs which achieved engraftment survived over 3 months in open kennel conditions without development of opportunistic infections.

Graft-versus-host-disease and complications

No dogs developed typical signs of GvHD in the skin, liver or gastro-intestinal tract. However, auto-immune like syndromes occurred in 4 dogs, including myasthenia gravis with antibodies to myoneural junctions and focal polymyositis in one [10], and immune thrombocytopenia in three. These data suggest that abnormalities in the regulation of immunity may occur after fetal liver transplantation.

Discussion

Our data indicate that transplantation of cells from a single fetal liver can reconstitute hematopoiesis and immunity in lethally irradiated recipients; they also demonstrate that sufficient numbers of progenitor cells are present in a single canine fetal liver to restore hematopoiesis and relatively normal T- and B-cell function.

Recovery of hematopoiesis was rapid with complete restoration of peripheral blood counts and bone marrow cellularity within one month.

Immunologic recovery was comparatively delayed, but sufficient after the first 3 months to allow for prolonged survival free of opportunistic infections. Transplantation of fetal liver cells did not produce clinically apparent GvHD even when the donors of fetal liver cells were completely mismatched with the recipients for DLA antigens. Antibody mediated autoimmune like syndromes (myasthenia gravis and immune thrombocytopenia) were observed supporting the abnormal regulation of B-cell function. Similar disorders have been reported following bone marrow transplantation.

Engraftment was reliably obtained for DLA-matched transplants with high-dose TBI alone. Failure of engraftment was a major problem, however, for recipients of DLA-mismatched fetal liver cells. We and others [11, 12] were unable to overcome this problem by high-dose total body irradiation alone. Substantial engraftment could be achieved in many dogs, however, by combining high-dose TBI with pre- and post-transplant cyclosporine. Escalation in the dose of TBI to 16.1 Gy led to increased mortality due to non-hematopoietic toxicity and infections.

These data suggest that fetal liver may be an effective source of hematopoietic cells for transplantation in patients with hematologic or immunologic diseases, who lack an HLA-identical donor for bone marrow transplantation. Successful transplantation will require development of an effective yet tolerable immunosuppressive preparative regimen.

The dose of total body irradiation required for sustained engraftment of fetal liver cells is higher than that typically employed for MHC-identical bone marrow transplants. This may explain the high frequency of graft failure with human fetal liver cell transplants.

References

1. Grebe SC, Streilen JW: Graft-versus-host reactions: A review. Adv Immunol 22: 119–221, 1976
2. Korngold R, Sprent J: Features of T cells causing H-2 restricted lethal graft-versus-host disease across minor histocompatibility barriers. J Exp Med 155: 182, 1982
3. Beatty PG, Clift RA, Mickelson EM, et al.: Marrow transplantation from related donors other than HLA-identical siblings. N Engl J Med 313: 765–71, 1985
4. Champlin RE, Gale RP: Hematopoiesis and immune reactivity of human fetal liver cells. In: Lucarelli G, Fliedner TM, Gale RP (eds) Fetal Liver Transplantation, Amsterdam, Excerpta Medica, 1980, pp 117–125
5. Uphoff DE: The preclusion of secondary phase of irradiation syndrome by innoculation of fetal hematopoietic tissue following total body irradiation. J Nat Cancer Inst 20: 625, 1958
6. Publication of the Radiobiological Institute of the Organization for Health Research TNO, Rijswijk (ZH), The Netherlands, 1975
7. Gale RP, Touraine JL, Lucarelli G (eds): Fetal Liver Transplantation, Alan R Liss Inc, New York, 1985
8. O'Reilly RJ, Pollack MS, Kapoor N, et al.: Fetal liver transplantation in man and animals. In: Gale RP (ed) Recent advances in Bone Marrow Transplantation. Alan R Liss, Inc, New York, 1983, 799–830

18

9. Stitzel KA, Champlin RE, Gale RP: Fetal liver transplantation: a possible alternative to bone marrow as a source of hematopoietic cells for transplantation. In: Gale RP (ed) Recent Advances in Bone Marrow Transplantation. Alan R Liss, Inc, New York, 1983, pp 29–38

10. Champlin R, Cain G, Stitzel K, Gale RP: Fetal liver cell transplantation in dogs: Results with DLA-compatible and incompatible grafts. In: Gale RP, Touraine JL, Lucarelli G (eds) Fetal Liver Transplantation, Alan R Liss Inc, New York, 1985, 195–204

11. Cain GC, Cardimet GN, Cuddon PC, Gale RP, Champlin RE: Myasthenia gravis and polymyositis in a dog following fetal hematopoietic cell transplantation. Transplantation 1985 (in press)

12. Saltzstein EC, Bortin MM, Rimm AA: Long lived canine allogeneic radiation chimera produced with combined fetal liver and thymus cells. Transplant 18: 461–2, 1974

13. Thomas ED, Collins JA, Kasakura S: Lethally irradiated dogs given infusions of fetal and adult hematopoietic tissue. Transplant 1: 514–20, 1963

Thymus 10:19–31 (1987)

Variation of treatment conditions alters the outcome of fetal liver transplantation in dogs

OTTO PRÜMMER, WENCESLAO CALVO and THEODOR M. FLIEDNER

Department of Clinical Physiology and Occupational Medicine, University of Ulm, D-7900 Ulm, FRG

Key words: fetal liver transplantation, dog, hematopoiesis, immune functions, graft-versus-host disease

Summary. Fetal liver transplants (FLT) were carried out in 25 beagles under various conditions. Graft recipients were prepared with fractionated total body x-irradiation (TBI) of 3 × 6 Gy or 2 × 6 Gy and rescued with cryopreserved fetal liver cells (FLC) from 51- to 52-day-old or 43- to 46-day-old, DLA-identical siblings or DLA-haploidentical, homozygous half-siblings. In all groups, FLC grafts contained comparable numbers of granulocyte-macrophage progenitor cells. Initial engraftment was achieved in all dogs. However, low TBI dose and DLA haplotype disparity between donor and recipient were associated with graft failure in 1/3 and 2/9 recipients, respectively, within 10–16 days of treatment. Lectin-responsive host type lymphocytes circulated for more than 5 weeks, whereas bone marrow metaphases were always of donor sex. Reduced TBI dose and young donor age were associated with delayed granulocyte recovery. Moreover, circulating platelets and total lymphocytes as well as T and B-cell numbers and rose more slowly in recipients of immature FLC grafts than in the other groups. Delayed cutaneous hypersensitivity reactions were normal one year after FLT, whereas the IgM component of the hemagglutinin response to sheep red blood cells was depressed. In mixed leukocyte culture, chimeric lymphocytes were tolerant to host antigens. Nonetheless, clinical and histological signs compatible with low-grade graft-versus-host disease were recorded in 10 or 25 animals. Thus FLT in dogs could be carried out, even across DLA barriers, without severe graft-versus-host disease. However, a low pretransplant TBI dose, incomplete DLA match and young age of the fetal donor were associated with graft rejection and protracted restoration of hemopoiesis and immune functions.

Introduction

The liver of mammalian embryos and fetuses is the primary hemopoietic organ during certain stages of development [6]. Fetal liver cells (FLC) of appropriate gestational ages are rich in hemopoietic stem cells but contain few, if any, postthymic T cells [9]. Accordingly, allogeneic FLC may restore hemopoiesis and, to a lesser degree, immune functions without severe acute graft-versus-host disease (GvHD) when transplanted between strongly histoincompatible mouse strains [7, 8, 13, 30].

The dog has frequently been used as an experimental animal in hemopoietic stem cell transplantation studies [31]. However, FLT was rarely

Address for offprints: Dr. Otto Prümmer, Dept. of Clinical Physiology and Occupational Medicine, University of Ulm, Oberer Eselsberg M 24, D-7900 Ulm, FRG.

carried out in this outbred species. Limited experience indicates that, if engraftment is achieved, FLC may restore hemopoiesis and immune reactivity without life-threatening GvHD [3, 15–17, 25, 16]. This communication briefly reviews our experience with canine FLT and describes the influence of treatment variables such as host conditioning, donor age, and histocompatibility between donor and recipient on the outcome of FLT.

Materials and methods

Animals

Beagles aged 7–15 months and weighing 10.2–19.0 kg were used throughout this study. Animals had been dewormed and vaccinated against parvovirus, distemper, hepatitis, leptospirosis, and rabies prior to entering the study.

Fetal liver transplantation

All aspects of the transplantation procedure have been described in detail elsewhere [15]. Briefly, fetuses that were genetically homozygous for dog leukocyte antigens (DLA)-A, B, and D were obtained by partial or total hysterectomy 43–52 days after mating. Single cell suspensions from fetal liver were cryopreserved under liquid nitrogen [5] until use. Twenty-five graft recipients were prepared with 3×6 Gy (days -4, -2, and 0) or 2×6 Gy (days -2 and 0) total body x-irradiation (TBI) and subsequently intravenously infused (day 0) with FLC from DLA-identical siblings or DLA-haploidentical half-siblings of various gestational ages (Table 1). Similar numbers of granulocyte-macrophage progenitor cells (CFU–GM) per kg recipient body weight were administered in all groups, although mononuclear cell numbers were higher in group 3 than in groups 2, 4, and 5. After death of the animals, complete autopsies were performed. Most data of group 1 have been reported previously [15–17]. Therefore, the present article is mainly concerned with observations in groups 2–5.

Table 1. Data on dogs given fetal liver cell grafts from DLA-identical siblings or DLA-haploidentical half-siblings.

Hosts		Irradiation dose (Gy)	Grafts			
Group	n		Gestation[a] day	DLA	MNC/kg ($\times 10^{-8}$)	CFU–GM/kg ($\times 10^{-4}$)
1	10	3×6	52	ident.	0.5 (0.2–1.6)[b]	4.8 (0.9–19.8)
2	3	2×6	51	ident.	0.2 (0.1–0.5)	7.3 (6.1–17.0)
3	3	3×6	45	ident.	1.2 (1.1–1.4)	8.0 (6.3–9.8)
4	5	3×6	51	haploid.	0.2 (0.2–0.4)	7.1 (5.9–7.5)
5	4	3×6	43–46	haploid.	0.4 (0.2–0.4)	7.2 (4.7–11.6)

[a] Day after mating.
[b] Median (range).

Routine hematology

Complete blood counts, including reticulocyte and platelets counts, were performed three times before and at intervals after transplantation by routine methods [15]. Bone marrow was aspirated from the iliac crest and morphologically evaluated on smears stained with May-Grunwald-Giemsa.

Culture of CFU–GM and assessment of stimulating serum activities

Granulocyte-macrophage colony-forming cells in blood and bone marrow were quantitated in 7-day agar cultures as described previously [16]. Serum levels of colony-stimulating activity were estimated according to the number of CFU–GM stimulated by the respective test serum from a CFU–GM-rich mononuclear blood cell population [16]. Serum endotoxin levels were quantitated with a sensitive limulus lysate assay.

Lymphocyte subpopulations

Surface immunoglobulins (sIg) on peripheral blood mononuclear cells (PBMC) were stained in direct immunofluorescence with a polyclonal goat-antidog Ig antibody (rhodamine-conjugated $F(ab')_2$ fragments; Cappel Laboratories, Cochranville) [18]. Surface Ig-positive lymphocytes were scored as B-cells. Lymphocytes with a dot-like distribution of the acid α-naphthyl acetate esterase (ANAE) were scored as ANAE-positive [18, 35]. ANAE-positivity has been reported to be a canine T-cell marker [35]. In groups 4 and 5, lymphocytes expressing the canine equivalent of Thy-1 were identified with the mouse monoclonal antibody F3-20-7 [11] (generous gift from Dr. W. Buurman, Maastricht) and visualized with the rhodamine-conjugated $F(ab')_2$ fragments of a polyclonal goat-antimouse Ig antibody (Cappel) in indirect immunofluorescence. In normal dogs, about 70% (50–85%) of blood lymphocytes were Thy-1-positive.

Serum immunoglobulins

Serum levels of immunoglobulins (IgG, IgM, and IgA) were quantitated by single radial immunodiffusion (RID-Kit dog IgG, IgM, IgA; Miles Laboratories, Elkhart).

Lymphocyte transformation

The lymphocyte transformation (LT) assay has been described previously [18]. Briefly, 5×10^4 PBMC were stimulated in round-bottomed microwells with optimal concentrations of phytohemagglutinin (PHA) (2.5 μg/ml), concanavalin A (Con A) (20 μg/ml), or pokeweed mitogen (PWM) (2 μl/ml) for four days in supplemented Waymouth medium. Cryopreserved PBMC from individual dogs obtained before and after transplantation were tested in single experiments. For the last 18–20 h of culture, ^{3}H-thymidine was added and incorporated activity was assessed by liquid scintillation counting. Results were expressed as mean counts per minute (cpm) of triplicate determinations.

Mixed leukocyte culture

In mixed leukocyte cultures (MLC), 5×10^4 PBMC from the test animal were stimulated with 5×10^4 irradiated (20 Gy), DLA-incompatible PBMC for 5 days under identical conditions as described for the LT assay [18]. Proliferative activity was assessed by liquid scintilation counting. In tolerance tests, PBMC of the chimera were stimulated with cryopreserved PBMC of the host, with autologous PBMC, and with allogeneic PBMC from DLA-identical and DLA-nonidentical donors.

Delayed cutaneous hypersensitivity

About one year after FLT, long-term survivors of groups 1, 2, and 4 were subcutaneously inoculated at the hind leg with 1 ml of a trivalent vaccine containing distemper virus, hepatitis virus, and leptospira antigens (Candur SHL; Behringwerke, Marburg). Four weeks later, animals were challenged intradermally at the outer side of the ear with 0.1 ml of the vaccine. Controls were carried out with the solvent or with saline. At the inoculation site, the thickness of the ear was measured with a screw micrometer before and at 48 h and 72 h after challenge. The increase was assessed both in absolute and in relative terms.

Antibody response to sheep red blood cells

At the day of vaccination with Candur SHL, long-term survivors were intravenously injected with 2 ml of a 20% sheep red blood cell (SRBC) solution in saline. Serum samples were obtained before and at intervals for four weeks after inoculation and kept frozen until use. Serum was inactivated (30 min at 56 °C) and incubated for another hour with phosphate-buffered saline (PBS) 5×10^{-3} M dithiothreitol (DTT) to distinguish between total and DTT-labile (IgM) antibodies [1]. Hemagglutinating antibodies were detected by incubating 50 μl of serial two-fold dilutions of the test serum with 10 μl of SRBC in PBS (2×10^8 SRBC/ml) for 24 h at room temperature. Then plates were tilted (45° angle) and read after 3 min. The anti-SRBC titer was defined as $-\log_2$ of the last serum dilution that prevented SRBC from streaming down the bottom of the well. For the evaluation of the secondary response, the whole procedure was repeated 10 weeks after the primary inoculation.

Results

Engraftment and survival

In all 25 FLC recipients, an initial engraftment with foci of hemopoiesis in bone marrow aspirates and rising blood cell counts was noted. Whereas there was a permanent take in all ten animals in group 1, reduction of the conditioning TBI dose ($2 \times 6\,\mathrm{Gy}$) or transfer of homozygous, DLA-haploidentical FLC resulted in secondary rejections with declining blood granulocyte counts 10–16 days after grafting in 1/3 (group 2), 1/5 (group 4), and 1/4 (group 5) dogs, respectively (Table 2). During the final rejection phase, blood lymphocyte numbers always exceeded the granulocyte counts. A second and third transplant failed to engraft after corticosteroid treatment in one animal of group 5. Thirteen dogs had to be killed between days 57 and 223 owing to progressive weight loss, which most likely was a consequence of pancreatic fibrosis and exocrine insufficiency of the organ. In a few cases, septicemia, pneumonia, jaundice, or ascites complicated the condition. Nine long-term survivors are alive or were killed between one and two years after FLT owing to lack of kennel space.

Erythropoiesis

There was no difference among the various groups with respect to the restoration of erythropoiesis. Normoblasts and reticulocytes appeared in the circulation after day 7 and attained peak values of 260 normoblasts/μl and 128×10^3 reticulocytes/μl between days 24 and 27 in groups 2–5. Within 2–3 weeks, cell counts dropped to normal or subnormal levels. As noted earlier in group 1 [15], erythrocyte counts and hemoglobin levels only transiently approached pretreatment values 5–6 weeks after FLT and were subnormal for one year thereafter.

Granulopoiesis and monocytopoiesis

Monocytes and granulocytes disappeared from the circulation within 5–7 days after the first TBI fraction and started to rise again 4–7 days after FLT. Monocyte numbers reached mean pretreatment values by day 19 irrespective of the treatment modality in groups 2–5. In contrast, granulocytes recovered more rapidly in recipients prepared with $3 \times 6\,\mathrm{Gy}$ and grafted with FLC from old fetuses (groups 1 and 4) than in the remaining animals (groups 2, 3, and 5) (Table 3). Mean pretreatment values were attained between days 20 and 33.

These differences were not reflected by the frequency of bone marrow or blood CFU–GM. Similar to findings in group 1 [16], low numbers of

Table 2. Graft rejection and survival after fetal liver transplantation.

Recipient group	Rejection	Survival (days)
1	0/10[a]	57–90 (n = 6); > 500 (n = 4)
2	1/3	*21*,[b] 598, 599
3	0/3	83, 90, 108
4	1/5	*19*, 68, 105, 508, 572
5	1/4	*28*, 76, 223, > 300

[a] Grafts rejected/total number of grafts.
[b] Underlined numbers denote animals that rejected their grafts.

Table 3. Granulocyte recovery in fetal liver cell recipients.

| Group | n^a | Granulocyte count $> 1 \times 10^9/l$ (day) | |
		Median	Range
1	10	11	9–13
2	2	13	–
3	3	14	14–15
4	4	11	10–11
5	3	13	12–13

[a] Number of animals with sustained engraftment.

bone marrow CFU–GM were detected 3 days after transplantation in groups 2–5, and their relative incidence remained normal after day 10 (Table 4). Significant numbers of circulating CFU–GM were first detected on day 7. After day 14, their incidence per ml blood was elevated for one year even under the treatment conditions of groups 2–5. Since splenic CFU–GM pools were severely depressed in most of the animals, extramedullary hemaopoiesis in the spleen could not account for the expanded pool of circulating progenitors. An early peak of the colony-stimulating activity in serum 3–7 days after FLT coincided with the initial recovery phase of granulopoiesis and monocytopoiesis and was not paralleled by elevated serum endotoxin levels.

Megakaryopoiesis

In bone marrow aspirates, megakaryocytes were normally detected on days 7 or 10 after FLT. Between days 5 and 14, 3.8 ± 1.4 ($\bar{x} \pm SD$) platelet transfusions had to be administered to keep platelet counts above $20 \times 10^9/l$. Recipients of mature FLC (groups 1, 2, and 4) had their platelet counts slightly faster restored than animals grafted with cells from younger fetuses (groups 3 and 5) (Table 5). Pretreatment levels were recorded 4–5 weeks after FLT.

Lymphocytes

Blood lymphocyte numbers recovered more slowly than noted for granulocytes and platelets. Until day 22, there was no difference among

Table 4. Restoration of CFU–GM after fetal liver transplantation.

| Time after grafting | n^a | CFU–GM ($\bar{x} \pm SE$) | |
		Per ml blood	Per 10^5 bone marrow MNC
Before FLT	35	35 ± 8	179 ± 11
Day 3	12	0 ± 0	14 ± 5
Day 10	12	13 ± 4	126 ± 23
Day 21	12	175 ± 38	182 ± 49
Day 370	4	86 ± 26	218 ± 37

[a] Number of determinations in recipients with sustained engraftment (groups 2–5).

Table 5. Platelet recovery in fetal liver cell recipients.

Group	n[a]	Platelet count $> 100 \times 10^9/l$ (day)	
		Median[b]	Range
1	10	20.5	17–25
2	2	22.5	21–24
3	3	22.0	22–25
4	4	21.5	21–22
5	3	23.0	23–24

[a] Number of animals with sustained engraftment.
[b] The common median for groups 1, 2, and 4 was day 21; for groups 3 and 5 day 23.

treatment groups. Afterwards, more mature FLC grafts (groups 2 and 4) were associated with a faster lymphocyte restoration than observed after transplantation of younger cells (groups 3 and 5). Normal values were reached by day 101 (groups 2 and 4) and by day 270 (groups 3 and 5). In the former groups, B-cells rose more rapidly than total lymphocytes and T cells. Normal B-cell counts were recorded by day 35, whereas ANAE-positive and Thy-1-positive lymphocytes attained mean pretreatment levels by days 75 and 101, respectively. No such difference among lymphocyte subpopulations was detected in groups 3 and 5. For about two months after FLT, part of the circulating lymphocytes were of host origin (Table 6), whereas proliferating bone marrow cells were always of donor sex.

In vitro blastogenesis

Proliferative responses after stimulation with PHA, Con A, and PWM, as well as after alloactivation in MLC were significantly depressed (two-sided U-test) for seven weeks after transplant in groups 3 and 4. Whereas the lectin responses were normal afterwards, MLC reactions tended to be impaired for 9 months. Thus LT and MLC results were comparable to the findings in group 1 [17]. In the two dogs of group 2 examined, blastogenesis was depressed at day 28 (LT) and until day 75 (MLC).

Table 6. Origin of Con A-responsive blood mononuclear cells after fetal liver transplantation.[a]

Days post-transplant	No. of animals	Percent host metaphases[b]	
		Median	Range
35–49	9	15	0–72
75–79	6	0	0–60
192–203	3	0	–
370	2	0	–

[a] Data from groups 3–5.
[b] Twenty to fifty metaphases were routinely evaluated.

Serum immunoglobulins

In groups 2, 4, and 5, serum levels of IgG, IgM, and IgA were followed. Nadir values were recorded on day 21 (IgM; 47% of control), days 21–35 (IgA; 43% of control) and day 49 (IgG; 63% of control). Pretreatment levels were reached by days 49–75 (IgM), day 131 (IgG), and day 192 (IgA). Thus the sequence of events resembled findings in group 1 [17] but IgM and IgG levels were subnormal for a longer time in the present study.

Delayed cutaneous hypersensitivity

Eight FLC recipients from groups 1, 2, and 4 were tested for skin reactivity about one year after FLT. Subsequent to vaccination with Candur SHL and challenge, the increase in ear thickness at the inoculation site was in the normal range and there was no difference among the treatment groups tested (Table 7).

Antibody response to sheep red blood cells

After inoculation of SRBC, the primary hemagglutination titer was lower in long-term survivors one year after FLT ($-\log_2 = 11.2 \pm 0.9$; $\bar{x} \pm$ SE) than in normal control dogs (16.3 ± 2.2). Since the DTT-resistant components were identical (FLC recipients, 7.8 ± 0.3; normal controls, 7.4 ± 0.7) in both groups, transplanted animals appeared to be deficient in their primary IgM response. After repeated inoculation, the total antibody titers were approached in FLC recipients (12.1 ± 0.8) and controls (14.0 ± 0.9), and there was no DTT-labile component detectable in graft recipients. In control dogs, the DTT-resistant antibody titer was still lower (9.0 ± 1.3) than the total hemagglutination titer.

Graft-versus-host disease

In 10 dogs killed between days 60 and 125 after FLT, mild skin or liver changes were observed clinically or histologically that were indistinguishable from low-grade GvHD. Lymphocytic infiltration of the intestinal

Table 7. Delayed cutaneous hypersensitivity in long-term survivors after fetal liver transplantation.[a]

	Ear thickness (mm)		Increase	
	0 h	48–72 h[b]	mm	%
FLC recipients (n = 8)	1.91 ± 0.20[c]	3.88 ± 0.89	1.97 ± 0.85	104 ± 43
Normal controls (n = 6)	2.04 ± 0.23	3.80 ± 0.49	1.76 ± 0.52	88 ± 30

[a] Data from groups 1, 2, and 4 obtained about one year after grafting.
[b] Time after challenge with Candur SHL vaccine.
[c] Mean ± SD.

mucosa was noted in one animal. The fibrotic pancreas remnant was infiltrated by mononuclear cells in several cases. However, no clearcut difference was found between recipients of DLA-identical and DLA-haploidentical grafts. Long-term survivors were free of alterations resembling GvHD. When tested in MLC, circulating lymphocytes of recipients given homozygous, DLA-haploidentical grafts were tolerant to host antigens both early and late after FLT (Table 8).

Discussion

The present study confirms earlier findings [15–17] indicating that cryopreserved canine FLC are a potent source of pluripotent hemopoietic stem cells able to restore hemopoiesis and immune functions in adult recipients previously rendered aplastic by high-dose TBI. Dissimilar to observations after the transfer of DLA-identical sibling FLC obtained 52 days postconception, altered experimental conditions such as reduced TBI dose or DLA disparity between donor and recipient were associated with graft rejection in a number of cases. Residual, relatively radioresistant host cells recognizing minor histocompatibility antigens of the donor were likely to act as effector cells. This view is supported by the presence of lectin-responsive host lymphocytes in the circulation and the lymphocytic predominance among leukocytes during the final rejection phase in the present study. In man, T-cell-depleted, HLA-identical or HLA-mismatched, allogeneic bone marrow cells may fail to engraft durably, whereas graft failure is seldom observed with untreated, HLA-identical bone marrow [10, 29]. It is though that mature donor T-cells facilitate sustained engraftment by suppressing or eliminating residual host effector cells or by providing an helper activity for the growth of hemopoietic stem cells [10]. Accordingly, FLC that contain few mature T-lymphocytes [14] are at high risk to be rejected. This is particularly true in cases where immune reactivity of the host is insufficiently suppressed or where DLA disparity exists

Table 8. Tolerance of lymphocytes from FLC chimeras to host antigens in mixed leukocyte culture.

Responder		Stimulator[a]			
Chimera (AA)[b]	Day after FLT	Chimera (AA)	Host (AB)	Control 1 (AA)	Control 2 (CD)
179	74	0.7 ± 0.2[c]	0.5 ± 0.1	0.5 ± 0.1	3.9 ± 0.7
181	194	1.5 ± 0.1	2.8 ± 0.5	2.9 ± 0.5	38.0 ± 3.2
140	370	0.4 ± 0.2	0.5 ± 0.2	0.3 ± 0.1	11.0 ± 1.2
146	370	3.1 ± 0.6	5.0 ± 1.0	4.1 ± 2.0	52.0 ± 8.6

[a] Irradiated with 20 Gy.
[b] DLA-haplotype combination; heterozygous hosts were grafted with FLC from homozygous donors compatible for one DLA haplotype.
[c] Mean cpm ± SD ($\times 10^{-3}$) of triplicate determinations.

between donor and host [4, 32]. Spontaneous inactivation of CFU–GM by blood mononuclear cells [19] failed to reveal a higher sensitivity of fetal progenitor cells in comparison with adult bone marrow CFU–GM [20]. However, the inherent sensitivity of pluripotent stem cells to host effector cells may be different.

A large body of experimental evidence in rodents indicates that GvHD after allogeneic FLT is moderate and protracted, the severity depending on the genetic disparity between donor and recipient strains [7, 8, 13, 30]. Likewise, canine FLC may be transplanted into DLA-identical and non-identical hosts without severe GvHD [15, 17, 25, 27]. This findings were confirmed in the present study. However, in a number of recipients, gross skin changes or histological abnormalities in skin, liver, or the gastrointestinal tract were noted that were compatible with the presence of a moderate form of GvHD. Interestingly, there was no obvious difference between recipients of DLA-matched or haplotype-mismatched or between young and old grafts. This might reflect the limited number of experiments carried out or the low GvHD-causing potential of the respective grafts as a consequence of their insignificant contamination by mature T-cells. In addition, part of the alterations suggesting GvHD might have been produced by mechanisms different from classical, T-cell-mediated, acute GvHD, such as imbalance of immune regulation or viral infection [24, 26, 28]. Pancreatic fibrosis is a likely consequence of TBI in dogs [23, 33]. It is unclear whether mononuclear cell infiltrates after FLT represented the morphological equivalent of a pancreas-directed GvH reaction or merely reflected a secondary phenomenon subsequent to radiation-induced cell death and/or a peculiar homing pattern of the fetal liver-derived lymphocytes.

The lack of severe GvHD in FLC recipients could have reflected prolonged immune deficiency or tolerance of donor-derived lymphocytes to host antigens. Tolerance to host antigens was suggested by MLC experiments in which chimeric lymphocytes failed to respond to stored host cells but reacted readily to incompatible, allogeneic stimulators. In contrast, immune deficiency was an unlikely cause, since circulating lymphocytes recovered more rapidly in the present study than in beagles treated with 3×6 Gy TBI and comparable numbers of CFU–GM from autologous blood or bone marrow [18]. In addition, chimeric blood lymphocytes responded normally to lectin activation 2–3 months after FLT and skin reactivity was normal by one year. In spite of restored serum immunoglobulin levels and a rapid B-cell reconstitution, humoral immune functions were partially defective for at least one year. However, whereas the IgG response was found to be subnormal after bone marrow transplantation in man and dogs [1, 12, 34], the IgM component of the antibody response to SRBC was depressed in our FLC recipients.

After FLT in mice, proliferative B-cell functions manifest earlier than

T-cell functions [21]. This is in accordance with the rapid restoration of circulating B-cell numbers in recipients of liver grafts from fetuses older than gestation day 50 in the present study. The protracted recovery of total lymphocytes and T-cells may reflect an inductive function of the fetal liver for canine B-cell maturation and differentiation as is the case in mice [22]. Alternatively, host factors like persistence of radio-resistant B-cells [34] or deficient thymus function [2] may be involved. An expanded pool of total [14] and probably more differentiated lymphocytes in livers of older fetuses might also account for the hastened lymphocyte reconstitution in recipients of these FLC as compared with animals treated with cells from younger donors. However, even high lymphocyte proportions among blood leukocyte suspensions provided only a limited repopulation advantage when compared with bone marrow cells in autologous canine transplants [18]. Likewise, T-cell depletion from human bone marrow was associated with only a minor delay in lymphocyte recovery [10].

In the present study, all hemopoietic parameters depicted the same characteristics as noted earlier [15–17]. Although erythropoiesis predominated in fetal livers, monocytes and granulocytes were the most rapidly rising blood elements after grafting. Likewise, CFU–GM pools in blood and bone marrow were completely restored soon after FLT. Moreover, the small CFU–GM pool in the spleen excluded a causative role of splenic hemopoiesis for the high number of circulating CFU–GM. However, young donor age and reduced TBI dose were associated with protracted granulocyte and platelet recovery. It is likely that the same mechanisms that accounted for graft failure, i.e., residual host effector cells or lack of appropriate help by donor T-cells or a combination of both mechanisms were involved. Young fetal liver grafts contain less lymphocytes than older ones and thus appear to be more vulnerable.

In summary, canine FLC of various gestational ages proved capable of restoring hemopoiesis and immune functions in adult recipients compatible for at least one DLA haplotype that had been prepared with high-dose TBI. Even across a DLA-haplotype barrier no severe GvHD was induced. However, young donor age, DLA disparity between donor and recipient, and low TBI dose were associated with graft rejection or protracted recovery of hemopoiesis and immune reactivity. Thus, in several aspects, canine FLT resembles the transplantation of T-cell-depleted bone marrow in man and may serve as a preclinical model for the analysis of complications associated with the transfer of hemopoietic stem cell grafts lacking mature T-cells.

Acknowledgements

We thank all members of the Department of Clinical Physiology and Occupational Medicine, University of Ulm, who contributed to the

30

present study. The help of Dr. B. Kuhnt with part of the hysterectomies and of Dr. X. Zenzig with the assessment of serum endotoxin levels is gratefully acknowledged. Supported by the Deutsche Forschungsgemeinschaft, SFB 112, and the Radiation Protection Programme of the Commission of the European Communities, Contract BIO-C 345-80-D.

References

1. Abb J, Kolb HJ, Rodt HV, Grosse-Wilde H, Rieder I, Thierfelder S (1977) In vitro an in vivo immune response to specific antigens in canine marrow graft recipients. Z Immun-Forsch 158:152–161
2. Bödey B, Calvo W, Prümmer O, Carbonell F, Fliedner TM (1984) Regeneration of thymus after total body irradiation in dogs rescued with transfusion of fetal liver cells (Abstract). Exp Hematol 12:451
3. Champlin RE, Stitzel KA, Gale RP (1982) Fetal liver cell transplantation (FLCT) in dogs (Abstract). Exp Hematol 10, Suppl 10:31
4. Deeg HJ, Storb R, Shulman HM, Weiden PL, Graham TC, Thomas ED (1982) Engraftment of DLA-nonidentical unrelated canine marrow after high-dose fractionated total body irradiation. Transplantation 33:443–446
5. Fliedner TM, Körbling M, Calvo W, Bruch C, Herbst E, Fache I, Rüber E (1977) Cryopreservation of blood mononuclear leukocytes and stem cells in a large fluid volume: A preclinical model for a blood stem cell bank. Blut 35:195–202
6. Kelemen E, Calvo W, Fliedner TM (1979) Atlas of human hemopoietic Development. Berlin: Springer-Verlag
7. Löwenberg B (1975) Fetal liver transplantation. Publication of the Radiobiological Institute TNO, Rijswijk
8. Löwenberg B (1985) Fetal liver transplantation. In: Van Bekkum DW, Löwenberg B (eds) Bone marrow Transplantation: Biological Mechanisms and clinical Practice. New York: Marcel Dekker, pp 383–407
9. Lucarelli G, Fliedner TM, Gale RP (eds) (1979) Fetal liver Transplantation: Current Concepts and future Directions. Amsterdam: Excerpta Medica
10. Martin PJ, Hansen JA, Buckner D, Sanders JE, Deeg HJ, Stewart P, Appelbaum FR, Clift R, Fefer A, Witherspoon RP, Kennedy MS, Sullivan KM, Flournoy N, Storb R, Thomas ED (1985) Effects of in vitro depletion of T-cells in HLA-identical allogeneic marrow grafts. Blood 66:664–672
11. McKenzie JL, Fabre JW (1981) Studies with a monoclonal antibody on the distribution of Thy-1 in the lymphoid and extracellular connective tissues of the dog. Transplantation 31:275–282
12. Ochs HD, Storb R, Thomas ED, Kolb HJ, Graham TC, Mickelson E, Parr M, Rudolph RH (1974) Immunologic reactivity in canine marrow graft recipients. J Immunol 113:1039–1057
13. O'Reilly RJ, Pollack MS, Kapoor N, Kirkpatrick D, Dupont B (1983) Fetal liver transplantation in man and animals. In: Gale RP (ed) Recent Advances in bone marrow Transplantation. New York: Alan R Liss, pp 799–830
14. Prümmer O, Calvo W, Fliedner TM, Nothdurft W (1983) Immunological characterization of canine fetal liver cells. In: Gale RP (ed) Recent Advances in bone marrow Transplantation. New York: Alan R Liss, pp 841–848
15. Prümmer O, Raghavachar A, Werner C, Calvo W, Carbonell F, Steinbach I, Fliedner TM (1985) Fetal liver transplantation in the dog. I. Restoration of hemopoiesis with cryopreserved fetal liver cells from DLA-identical siblings. Transplantation 39:349–355
16. Prümmer O, Werner C, Raghavachar A, Nothdurft W, Calvo W, Steinbach KH, Fliedner TM (1985) Fetal liver transplantation in the dog. II. Repopulation of the granulocyte-macrophage progenitor cell compartment by fetal liver cells from DLA-identical siblings. Transplantation 40:498–503
17. Prümmer O, Calvo W, Werner C, Carbonell F, Fliedner TM (1985) Hemopoiesis and immune functions in dogs following fetal liver transplantation. In: Gale RP, Touraine J-L, Lucarelli G (eds) Fetal Liver Transplantation. New York: Alan R Liss, pp 175–194

18. Prümmer O, Raghavachar A, Fliedner TM 1985) Recovery of immune functions in dogs after total body irradiation and transplantation of autologous blood or bone marrow cells. Exp Hematol 13:891–898
19. Prümmer O, Nothdurft W, Fliedner TM, Baur G, Rüber E (1985) Canine blood mononuclear cells mediate contact-dependent impairment of granulocyte-macrophage colony formation by bone marrow cells. Exp Hematol 13:1033–1038
20. Prümmer O, Nothdurft W, Fliedner TM (1985) Canine blood mononuclear cells inhibit granulocyte-macrophage colony formation of adult bone marrow and fetal liver cells (Abstract). Blut 51:220
21. Rabinowich H, Umiel T, Globerson A (1983) T-cell progenitors in mouse fetal liver. Transplantation 35:40–48
22. Raff MC, Megson M, Owen JJT, Cooper MD (1976) Early production of intracellular IgM by B-lymphocyte precursors in mouse. Nature 259:224–226
23. Raghavachar A, Prümmer O, Fliedner TM, Calvo W, Steinbach IBE (1983) Stem cells from peripheral blood and bone marrow: a comparative evaluation of the hemopoietic potential in the dog. Int J Cell Cloning 1:191–205
24. Rappeport J, Reinherz E, Mihm M, Lopansri S, Parkman R (1979) Acute graft-versus-host disease in recipients of bone marrow transplants from identical twin donors. Lancet ii:717–720
25. Saltzstein EC, Bortin MM, Rimm AA, Hussey JL (1974) Long lived canine allogeneic radiation chimera produced with combined fetal liver and thymus cells. Transplantation 18:461–463
26. Snover DC (1985) Mucosal damage simulating acute graft-versus-host reaction in cytomegalovirus colitis. Transplantation 39:669–670
27. Stitzel KA, Champlin R, Gale RP (1983) Fetal liver transplantation in dogs: a possible alternative source of hematopoietic stem cells for transplantation. In: Gale RP (ed) Recent Advances in bone marrow Transplantation. New York: Alan R Liss, pp 831–840
28. Thein SL, Goldman JM, Galton DAG (1981) Acute 'graft-versus-host' disease after autografting for chronic granulocytic leukemia in transformation. Ann Intern Med 94:210–211
29. Trigg ME, Bozdech MJ, Sondel PM, Billing R, Finlay JL, Peterson AD, Stuiber M, Hong R (1984) Depletion of T-cells from mismatched allogeneic bone marrow: Results of transplantation in 23 patients with malignancy or aplastic anemia. Exp Hematol 12:412
30. Uphoff DE (1958) Preclusion of secondary phase of irradiation syndrome by inoculation of fetal hematopoietic tissue following lethal total-body x irradiation. J Natl Cancer Inst 20:625–632
31. Vriesendorp HM, van Bekkum DW (1980) Bone marrow transplantation in the canine. In: Shifrine M, Wilson FD (eds) The Canine as a biomedical research Model: Immunological, hematological and oncological Aspects. Technical Information Center, US Department of Energy, DOE/TIC-10 191, pp 153–202
32. Vriesendorp HM, Klapwyk WM, Heidt PJ, Hogeweg B, Zurcher C, van Bekkum DW (1982) Factors controlling the engraftment of transplanted dog bone marrow cells. Tissue Antigens 20:63–80
33. Vriesendorp HM, Zurcher C (1982) Late effects of total body irradiation in dogs treated with bone marrow transplantation. In: Fliedner TM, Gössner W, Patrick G (eds) Late Effects after therapeutic whole-body Irradiation. Report EUR 8070 EN. Commission of the European Communities, Luxembourg, pp 71–88
34. Witherspoon RP, Lum LG, Storb R (1984) Immunologic reconstitution after human marrow grafting. Sem Hematol 21:2–10
35. Wulff JC, Sale GE, Deeg HJ, Storb R (1981) Nonspecific acid esterase activity as a marker for canine T lymphocytes. Exp Hematol 9:865–870

Thymus 10:33–44 (1987)
© Martinus Nijhoff Publishers, Dordrecht   33

What kind of morphologically recognizable haemopoietic cells do we inject when doing foetal liver infusion in man?

ENDRE KELEMEN,[1] MARGIT JÁNOSSA,[1] WENCESLAO CALVO,[2]
THEODOR M. FLIEDNER,[2] MARGARET BOFILL[3] and GEORGE JANOSSY[3]

[1] 1st Department of Medicine, Semmelweis University Medical School, Budapest,
Hungary; [2] Abt. Klinische Physiologie u. Arbeitsmedizin, Universität Ulm/Donau, BRD;
[3] Department of Immunology, Royal Free Hospital Medical School, London, UK

Key words: developmental age, dyserythropoiesis, haemopoiesis, antenatal, human foetal liver, lymphoid-like cells, macrophages

Summary. There is no agreement, how to define the age of the embryo/foetus. — From the 15th (fertilization) week onwards the whole foetal liver contains some 10^9 free haemopoietic cells. Before, and up to the 30th–34th weeks, the liver is the main site of haemopoiesis. The differential of *embryonic* smears (up to wk 9) differs from that of *foetal* ones. The first invasion of circulating *primitive* erythroblasts seeding in the liver (early 5th wk) is accompanied by the appearance of a lot of sinusoidal *macrophages*. *Definitive* erythropoiesis expands during the 6th–7th wks. Granulocytic representation peaks at 15–16 wks. Megakaryocytes are small and have few nuclei/nuclear lobes. Five to 8, or even more per cent of single haemopoietic cells were *lymphoid-like* cells in the 5th–6th wk liver smear. These cells *precede* the development of any lymphoid structure in the foetus. Ordinary *lymphocytes* amount to less than 2% between 10 and 18 wks, and reached 3% at wk 24. — Percentage of *dyserythropoietic nuclei* in smears has been used to decide whether the injected cells could be regarded as 'physiological' cells. Ten out of 11 apparently healthy foetuses, delivered by hysterectomy/hysterotomy for maternal interest, aged $10\frac{1}{2}$ to $20\frac{1}{2}$ weeks, had mean 4.5% liver dyserythropoiesis. Extremely high dyserythropoiesis was associated with *multilineage,* instead of overwhelmingly erythroid haemopoiesis.

How to define the age of embryo/foetus: Disturbing lack of agreement

It is unfortunate that there is no agreement on how to define the age of the embryo/foetus. The widely used 'gestational age' could mean menstrual age (weeks since the 1st day of last menstrual period) or fertilization age (which is 2 weeks less than menstrual age). Absence of this distinction, in any work, may cause confusion. Developmental age, measuring the maximal length of long bones (instead of the measurement of the not sufficiently rigid crown-rump length) was recommended by us [10], at least between 8 to 22 *fertilization* weeks of age, but hitherto only few laboratories use this simple, well-reproducible method.

Address for offprints: Prof. Dr. Endre Kelemen, I. Belklinika, Korányi u 2/A, 1083 Budapest, Hungary.

Intrahepatic haemopoietic cell mass during the prevalence of liver haemopoiesis

The weight of the embryonic/foetal liver is less than 0.1 g at the 8th wk, about 1.0 g during the 10th wk, about 10.0 g at 16–18 wks, about 100.0 g at 30–32 wks, and 130–190 g at term.

The proportion of haemopoietic cells during the 5th wk is less than 10% of all cells found in the liver. They increase to 70% during the 8th wk, and remain at about this level until the 21st wk. Thereafter, haemopoietic cell representation slowly declines [7].

The total haemopoietic cell mass of the liver (on the basis of 100 samples) changes, as stated in following table:

Table 1.

$\sim 10^6$ at wk.	6 (fertiliz. age)
10^7	7
10^8	9–10
10^9	13–15
10^{10}	20–22[a]
10^9 at term	

[a] Peak values between the 21st and 28th wks. Before, and during this period the liver is the main site of haemopoiesis. From the 30th to 34th wks onward the calculated total haemopoietic cell mass of the whole marrow organ exceeds liver haemopoiesis (Figure 1).

Early haemopoietic cell differentials and the time of appearance of different kinds of cells. Macrophages. Primitive and definitive erythroblasts

The first invasion of circulating primitive erythroblasts seeding in the liver (end of the 4th and early 5th wks) is accompanied by the appearance of sinusoidal macrophages (Figure 2). The origin of these macrophages differs from later, marrow-derived ones. Figures 3–5 show the light and electron microscopic picture of these macrophage clusters. Up to 70% of the free intravascular cells observed in semithin sections of the liver of 4 and 4 1/2-wk-old embryos belonged to the macrophage series. Their number diminished abruptly during the weeks that followed, and at 9 wks only about 1% was found [9]. May-Grünwald-Giemsa stained smears from the liver of an embryo, around the time of starting extraembryonic to embryonic circulation, yielded (500 cells) 73.4% histiocytes/macrophages, 22.4% undefined, lymphoid-like blast cells (LLC), 2.4% small megakaryocytes, but only 1.4% primitive erythroblasts and 0.4% progranulocytes. The paucity of primitive erythroblasts appears to exclude the circulatory origin of these histiocytes/macrophages. Occasional erythropoietic islands were found in the sinusoidal vessels of the liver from the 6th wk onward [3, 8].

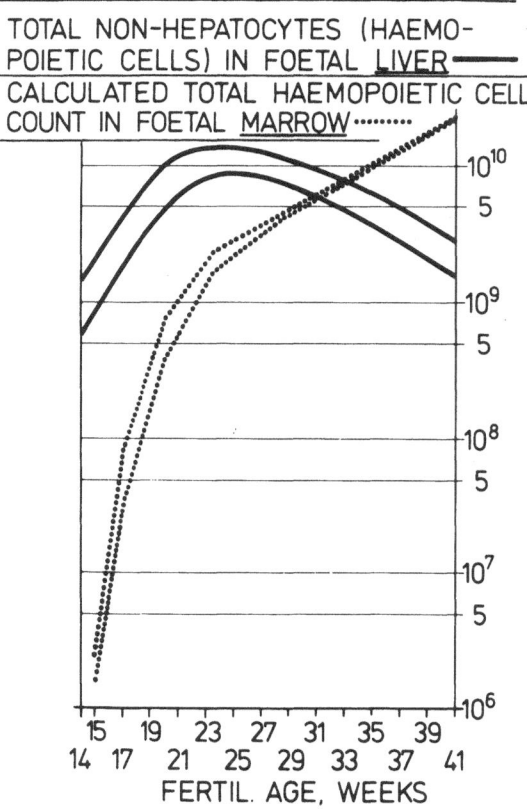

Figure 1. Calculated total haemopoietic cell counts in foetal liver (40 samples) and bone marrow (27 samples) from 15th wk of fertilization to term.

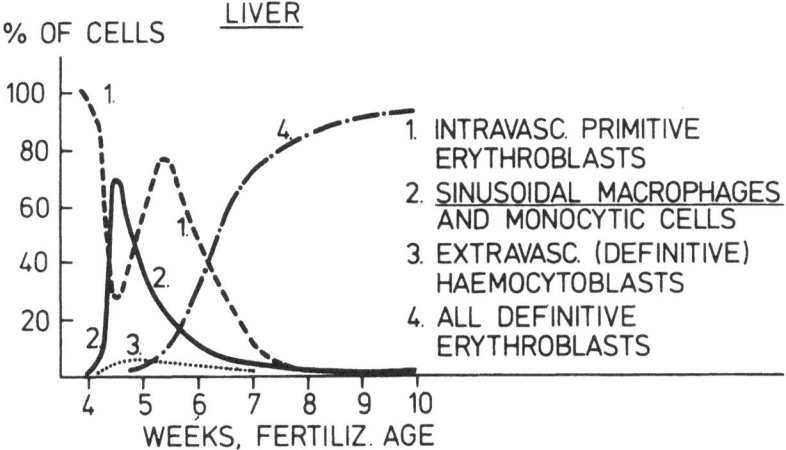

Figure 2. A pulse of sinusoidal macrophages and monocytic cells. Thirty-seven smears and 21 half-thin sections.

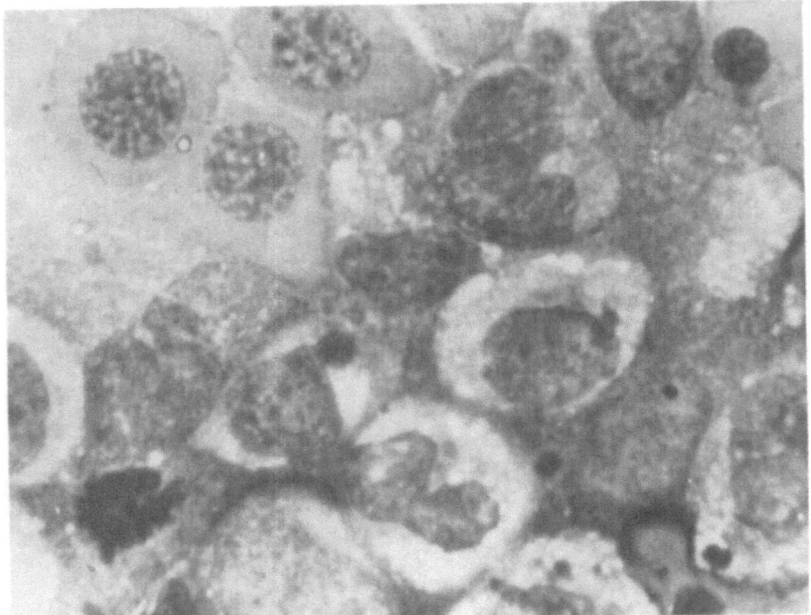

Figure 3. Light microscopic appearance of a macrophage cluster in a smear from a 6-wk-old embryonic liver. A few early, primitive erythroblasts are also shown beneath the monocytic cells (upper left).

The changing pattern of primitive and definitive erythroblasts is shown in Figure 6. Primitive erythroblasts derive from extrahepatic sources, whilst definitive erythroblasts originate from liver haemopoiesis. Figure 6 is a corrected version of a figure which appeared in [8]. We demonstrate that *expansion* of definitive erythropoiesis takes place already at wks 5–8

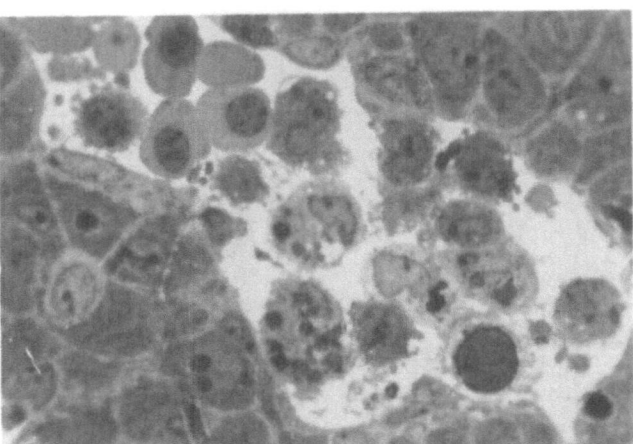

Figure 4. Half-thin section from the liver of a 5-wk-old embryo with intrasinusoidal accumulation of macrophages.

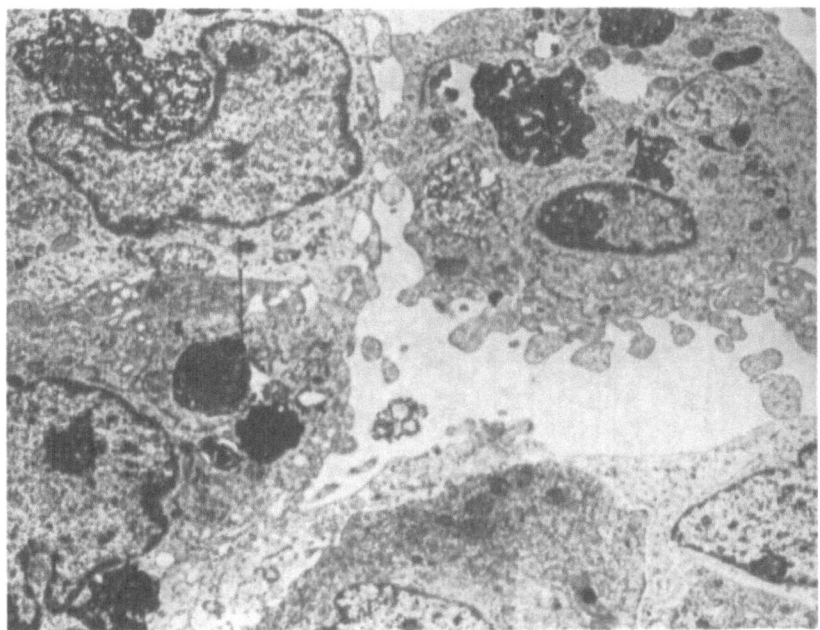

Figure 5. Electron microscopic picture from a macrophage cluster in the liver of a 5½-wk-old embryo.

in the liver, but only at wks 9–12 in the blood. This means that for up to 4 weeks the overwhelming majority of erythropoietic cells is *not released* from the liver. One could speculate that release of these blood cells could be connected with a relatively late event that *follows* morphological maturation.

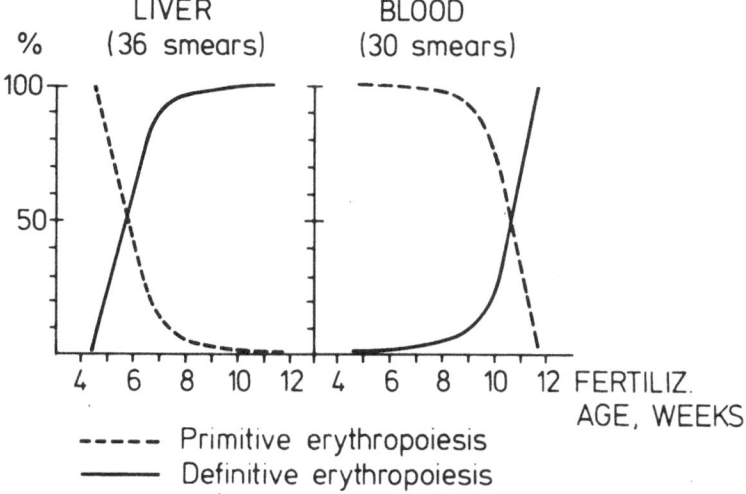

Figure 6. Changing pattern of primitive and definitive erythropoiesis in the embryonic/foetal liver and circulating blood.

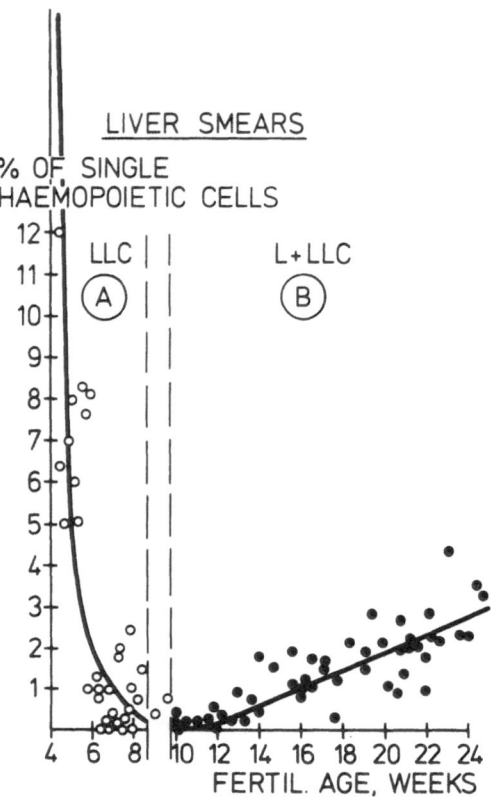

Figure 7. Per cent values of lymphoid-like cells (LLC, part A) and lymphocytes (L, part B) in embryonic/foetal liver smears.

Large, lightly-stained, benzidine-negative *haemocytoblasts* appear in the course of the 5th wk, amounting to less than 5% of extravascular cells (Figure 2). Pictures of haemocytoblasts were presented [7, 8].

Early lymphoid-like cells (LLC)

Five to 8, or even more per cent of single, intrahepatic haemopoietic cells were lymphoid-like cells in the 5th–6th wk liver smear, but the concentration of these cells diminished remarkably during the subsequent weeks and was less than 2% after the 6th week, and from this time onward they were not found in most smears. The nature of these cells — *preceding* the development of any lymphoid structure in the foetus — is now under our investigation. A part of these cells could, perhaps, represent certain levels of haemopoietic stem cells, and prethymic-T, or pre-B cells. We *failed* to identify these cells in methacrylate-embedded semithin sections. The changing concentration of these cells is demonstrated in Figure 7, and

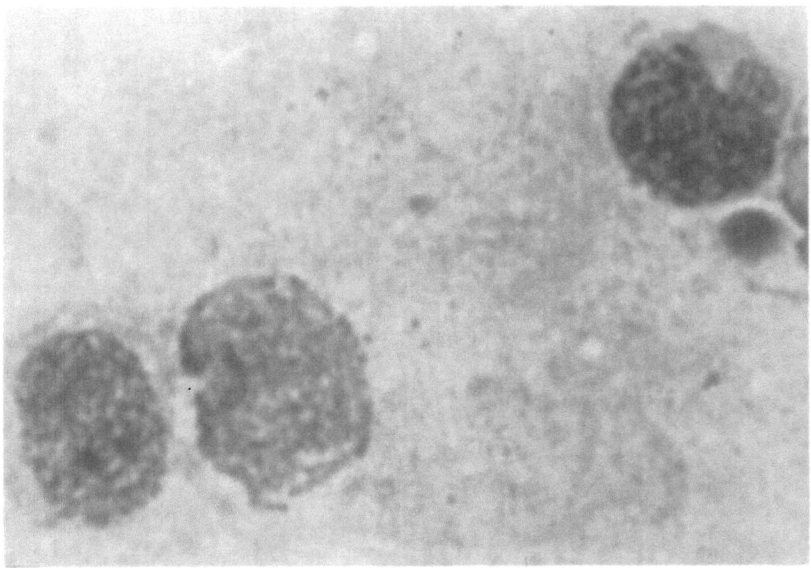

Figure 8. Undefined LLC-s in the liver smear of a 5-wk-old embryo. Coloured pictures of these and other cells of this embryonic liver were presented in [8] and [5].

their morphology is shown in Figure 8 [5]. It would be of interest *to explore* the possible beneficial effect of *embryonic* liver cell infusions, and compare it with that of the usually applied foetal ones. Among other differences, HLA-expression is reduced on the surface of these early embryonic cells. On the other hand, eventual *late* injurious effect(s) of *repeated* infusions should be considered in the future.

Ordinary lymphocytes

Ordinary lymphocytes are *absent,* or are *very rare* in 9–10 wk samples (less than 0.2%). Their concentration ranges between 0.2 and 1.0% between 11 to 16 wks, is between 1 and 2% in the course of 16–21 wks and between 2 and 3% of all free haemopoietic cells in smears from 21 to 25-wk-old foetuses (Figure 7). In the last years, more detailed analysis of the imm-unological systems, using monoclonal antibody techniques, has been car-ried out [1, 4].

Other systems: Time of appearance

Figure 9 contains some additional information as regards granulocytes and megakaryocytes and Table 2 surveys the time of appearance in the developing liver for each cell type, including parallel data on the emer-gence of different cells in the circulating blood.

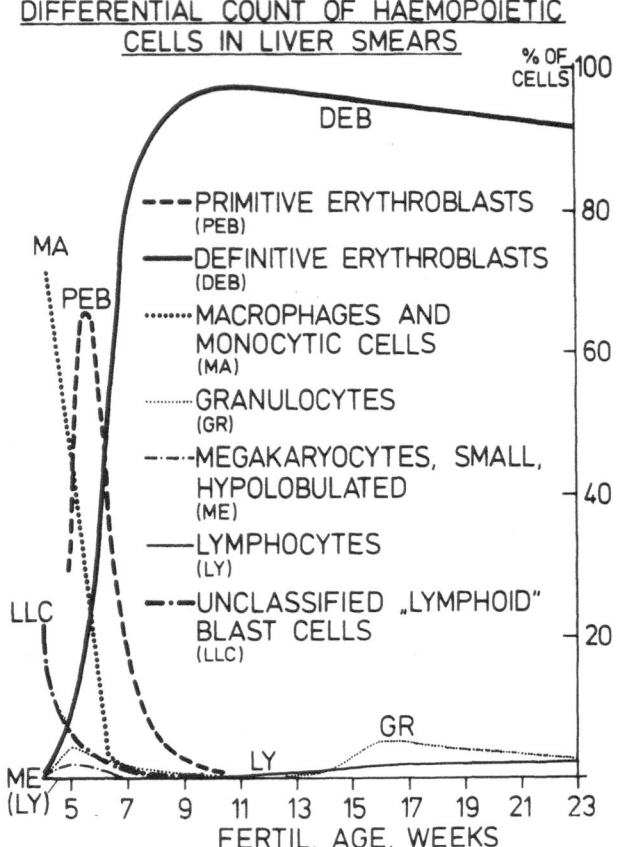

Figure 9. Demonstration of remarkable differences between the cell composition of embryonic *versus* foetal liver. In the embryonic phase lymphoid-like early progenitors (LLC), histiocytes/monocytic cells/macrophages (MA), and primitive erythroblasts (PEB) predominate. In the foetal period the overwhelming majority of liver haemopoietic cells are definitive erythroblasts (DEB). Lymphocytes and granulocytes appear in the foetal period. Foetal megakaryocytes — below 1% of haemopoietic cells — are not figured.

Non-recognizable progenitors

Although the outstanding significance of different uncommitted and committed stem cells is obvious, we did not deal with this subject in this morphokinetic presentation. Nevertheless, liver cells are 2 to 5 fold enriched for these progenitors as compared with bone marrow [12]. Pluripotent haemopoietic stem cells (CFU–GEMM) in the human foetal liver were found around wk 12, about 2–3 wks before their demonstrability in the marrow [2].

Liver dyserythropoiesis monitoring intrauterine stress

During the last 15 years we investigated more than 500 embryos/foetuses.

Table 2. Recognized first appearance of different blood cells in the prenatal human liver and blood.

	Liver	Blood
Lymphocyte-like cells[a]	4–5	. . . 4–5
Primitive erythroblasts[a]	4–5	3–4
Definitive erythroblasts[a]	4–5	7–8
Granuloblasts and early granulocytes[a]	5–6	6–8
Granulocytes, mature[a]	5–6	6–8
Macrophages/histiocytes[a]	4–5	3–4
Megakaryocytes[a]	4–5	4–5
Prethymic progenitors[b]	5–6	8–9
T-lymphocytes	10–12	10–12
Early pre-B cells[b]	6–7	8–9
B-lymphocytes	9–10	10–12
NK cells[b]	. . . 9–10	. . . 10–11

(numbers mean fertilization age in weeks.)
[a] *Before* established myeloid or lymphiod haemopoiesis
[b] *Before* established thymic or marrow haemopoiesis

In several instances it was not easy to decide whether the cells — that we eventually used to inject into recipients suffering from bone marrow aplasia — could be regarded as 'physiological' ones. Determination of the percentage of dyserythropoietic morphology in foetal liver smears has

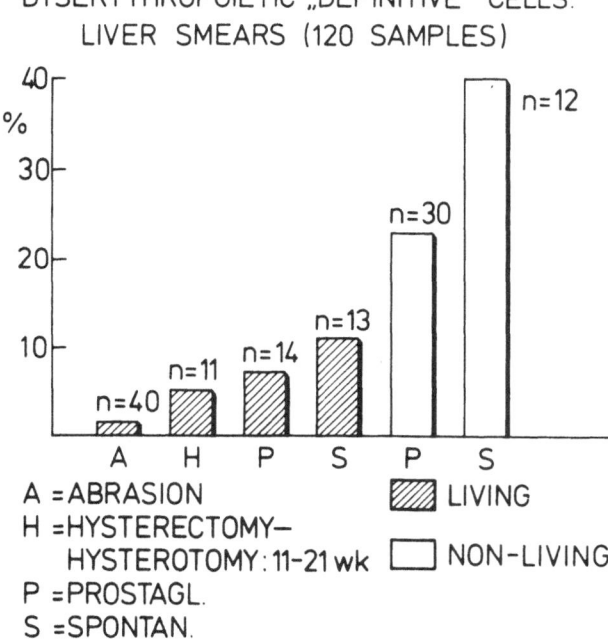

Figure 10. Liver dyserythropoiesis in relation with intrauterine stress. Three hundred to 500 nucleated red cells were counted in smears and the percentage of dyserythropoietic nuclei was calculated. 'Living' or 'not living' embryos or foetuses at the time of delivery.

42

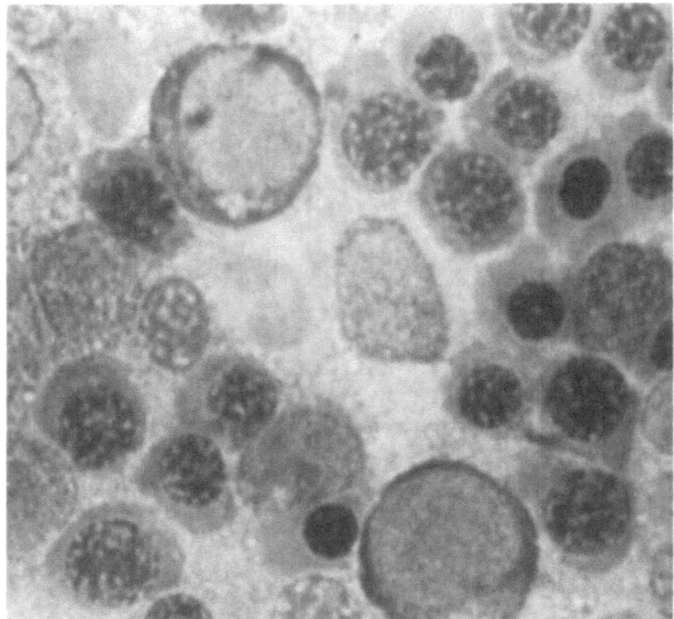

Figure 11. Normal (definitive) non-dyserythropoietic nuclear morphology in the liver.

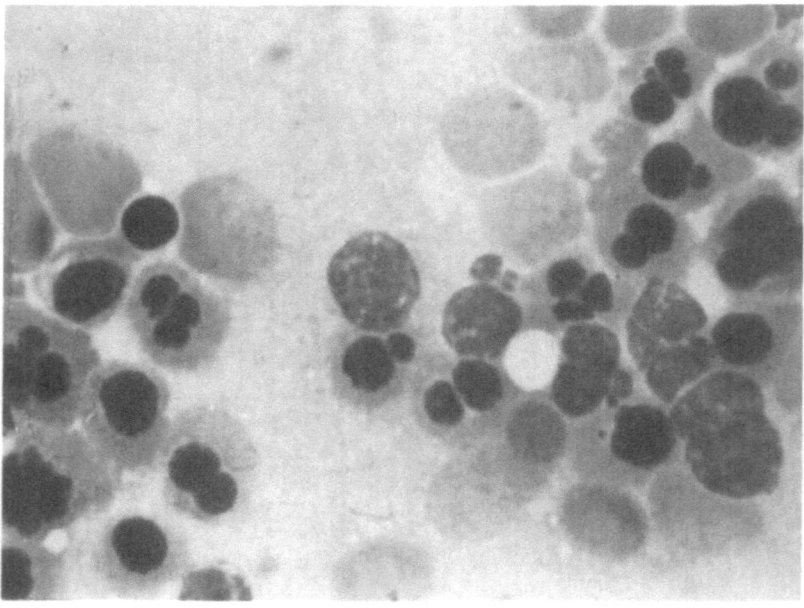

Figure 12.Pronounced liver dyserythropoiesis (over 50%) in a 13-wk-old foetus. The majority of (definitive) erythroblasts exhibits pathological nuclear morphology.

been used for this purpose in our laboratories [11]. As shown in Figure 10, the so-called 'physiological' dyserythropoiesis, if it exists, is very slight, especially in the embryo. During our studies, 11 apparently healthy foetuses, aged $10\frac{1}{2}$ to $20\frac{1}{2}$ wks, and deriving from mothers subjected to hysterectomy/hysterotomy were investigated immediately. Ten out of these selected samples had mean 4.5% liver dyserythropoiesis, and the highest value was 7.5%. Even these values might be, at least partly, connected with stress (surgery, anaesthesia)/hypoxia.

Work with Pajor, Zsolnay and Jánossa showed that substantially increased dyserythropoiesis, which characterizes spontaneous abortions, especially those with the delivery of non-living foetuses (see Figure 10) is, certainly, non-physiological. Samples with more than 10% dyserythropoiesis were excluded from therapeutic use. Owing to this exclusion, however, we cannot say, whether the infusion of such material would be less effective, or even injurious to the recipient.

Nevertheless, dyserythropoietic nuclei in 40% or more of intrahepatic red cells (in smears) were associated with *multilineal* — instead of overwhelmingly erythroid — heamopoiesis. The possible significance of this observation is subject of further investigation.

This paper is restricted to *our* work with *human* foetal liver and references to work of other groups are not included, even if related to the work of the authors.

References

1. Bofill M, Janossy G, Jánossa M, Burford GD, Seymour GJ, Wernet P, Kelemen E (1985) Human B cell development II. Subpopulations in the human fetus. J Immunol 134: 1531–1538
2. Hann IM, Bodger MP, Hoffbrand AV (1983) Development of pluripotent haematopoietic progenitor cells in the human fetus. Blood 62:118–123
3. Jánossa M, Kelemen E (1981) Erythroblastic islands in human extraembryonic and embryonic tissues. In: Hollán SR, Gárdos G, Sarkadi B (eds) Adv. Physiol. Sciences, Vol. 6. Genetics, Structure and Function of Blood Cells. Budapest: Akad. Kiadó, pp 81–83
4. Janossy G, Bofill M, Poulter LW, Rawlings E, Burford GD, Navarrette C, Ziegler A, Kelemen E: Separate ontogeny of two macrophage-like accessory cell populations in human fetus. J Immunol (in press)
5. Kelemen E (1974) Light microscopy of scattered unprocessed hemopoietic precursor cells in liver smears of a 6.35 mm crown-rump length human embryo. Exp Hematol 2:118–121
6. Kelemen E (1979) Small megakaryocytes in human embryonic liver. Blood Cells 5:101–102
7. Kelemen E, Calvo W (1982) Prenatal hematopoiesis in human bone marrow and its developmental antecedents. In: Trubowitz S, Davis S (eds) The Human Bone Marrow: Anatomy, Physiology and Pathophysiology, Vol I. Boca Raton: CRC Press, pp 3–41
8. Kelemen E, Calvo W, Fliedner TM (1979) Atlas of Human Hemopoietic Development. Berlin–Heidelberg–New York: Springer, pp 128–129

9. Kelemen E, Jánossa M (1980) Macrophages are the first differentiated blood cells formed in human embryonic liver. Exp Hematol 8:996–1000

10. Kelemen E, Jánossa M, Calvo W, Fliedner TM (1984) Developmental age estimated by bone-length measurement in human fetuses. Anat Rec 209:547–552

11. Pajor A, Kelemen E, Jánossa M (1983) Dyserythropoiesis magzati májban, mint a vetélés keltette stress intenzitásának jelzöje. Orv Hetil 124:619–622

12. Sieff CA, Emerson SG, Mufson A, Gesner TG, Nathan DG (1986) Dependence of highly enriched human bone marrow progenitors on hemopoietic growth factors and their response to recombinant erythropoietin. J Clin Invest 77:74–81

Thymus 10:45–56 (1987)
© Martinus Nijhoff Publishers, Dordrecht

Development of the immune system in human fetal liver

ROBERT PETER GALE

Department of Medicine, Division of Hematology and Oncology, UCLA School of
Medicine, Los Angeles, CA 90024, USA

Summary. Fetal liver is a major site of development of the human immune system. Pre-B and
B-lymphocytes are present in the human fetal liver at 12 weeks in a random distribution and
increase with gestation. Most fetal liver cells are pre-B but mature B-cells are also present.
Functional assays and transplantation experiments indicate that these B-cells are functional
and can transfer immunologic memory, albeit imperfectly, in fetal liver reconstituted recipients. T-cell development, in contrast, occurs predominantly in the thymus. Progenitors of
T-cells are present in fetal liver and can restore T-cell immunity in irradiated recipients.
Human fetal liver contains 1–2% mature T-cells; functional assays are likewise negative. NK
cells have been detected in human fetal liver at low frequency. Fetal liver also contains non-T,
non-B cells capable of suppressing the development of alloantigen reactive T-cells; these have
been termed veto cells. In summary, human fetal liver contains progenitors of several types
of lymphoid cells and is an important site of immune development. It also may play a role
in the induction of self tolerance during maturation of the immune system. These features
of fetal liver may have important implications for the success of fetal liver transplantation
in man.

Introduction

Fetal liver is a major site of immune development in man [1–6]. Lymphocytes are identifiable in human fetal liver at 6–7 weeks of gestation.
The proportion of lymphoid cells is variable, ranging between < 5% to
15% of the mononuclear, non-hepatic parenchymal cells. At this time the
fetal liver also contains substantial 'blast' cells, some of which may be
immature lymphoid cells or their progenitors. The proportion of lymphoid
cells is relatively constant until 20–24 weeks when they constitute > 20%
of mononuclear cells. The proportion of unidentifiable immature cells
gradually decreases during this period from 10% to < 2%.

B-lymphocyte development

Hematopoietic stem cells, probably arising from yolk sac progenitors and
possibly from other sites, migrate to the fetal liver after approximately 5
weeks of gestation. Under appropriate microenvironmental and probably
growth factor control, the cells differentiate to B-lymphocyte progenitors
[7–11] and eventually to mature B-cells. Pre-B cells, cells with identifiable
cytoplasmic heavy μ-chain $(c\mu^+)$, are the first readily detectable B-

lymphocytes in mammals [7]. Expression of $c\mu$ results from the productive rearrangement of V_H, D_H, J_H, $C\mu$ heavy chain genes from their germ-line configuration on one parental allele. This μ-chain probably has no hydrophobic tail (secreted type) explaining the absence of surface IgM. Next V_L, D_L, and C_L light chain genes are rearranged with synthesis of K or λ. μ-heavy chains of the membrane type are now produced, these combine with K or λ chains to form monomeric IgM which is displayed on the cell surface. δ chains are also synthesized at this time, possibly because of alternate splicing of a $\mu\delta$ mRNA and IgD appears on the cell surface. Switching to γ, ε and α heavy chain synthesis occurs via further genomic rearrangements with deletion of the $C\mu\delta$ segment with resultant expression of IgG, IgE or IgA. Because persistence of $\mu\delta$ mRNA, triplet cells with surface IgM, IgD and IgG or IgA are occasionally observed. Finally, mature B-cells differentiate to a plasma cell with subsequent loss of surface immunoglobulin (sIg) and secretion of Ig as a result of alternate processing of the heavy chain mRNA. A model of B-cell development is indicated in Figure 1, and is reviewed in reference [12].

Kamps and Cooper have reported detailed studies of B-cell development in human fetal liver [11]. They found 3–4% pre-B and B-cells in fetal livers of 12–15 weeks gestation. Pre-B cells had an immune phenotype of $\mu^+ K^- \lambda^-$ whereas B-cells were $\mu^+ K^+ \lambda^-$ or $\mu^+ K^- \lambda^+$ cells. The ratio of K to λ cells was similar to that observed in adults; 2 to 1. Pre-B and B-cells were randomly distributed throughout fetal liver and were not observed in relation to other hematopoietic cells or in clusters as occurs in the germinal centers of the avian Bursa of Fabricius. Kamps and Cooper found that B-cells tended to occur singly but occasional doublets or triplets were identified [11]. These multi-cell clusters contained both pre-B and B-cells but were restricted to a single isotype either $\mu^+ K^+$ or $\mu^+ \lambda^+$. These data are consistent with a model of in-situ development of B-cells in human fetal liver.

It is also possible to study B-cell development in fetal liver using monoclonal antibodies to B-cell related antigens [13–15]. Relevant antibodies are indicated in Figure 1. Most useful are antibodies to the common acute lymphoblastic leukemia antigen (CALLA), which reacts with early and mature B-cells, B1, which reacts with a wide range of immature and mature B-cells, B2, which reacts with more mature B-cells, RFB-1, which reacts with terminal deoxynucleotidyl transferase (TdT) positive cells but not pre-B or B-cells, and BA-1, which also reacts with TdT + cells. BA-1 has a pattern of reactivity similar to B1; it differs from RFB-1 by reacting with pre-B and B-cells. The relationship between B-cell development and antigen expression is shown schematically in Figure 1.

Rosenthal and coworkers reported detailed analyses of fetal liver cells using CALLA, B1 and B2 monoclonal antibodies [13]. These data are summarized in Table 1. They found approximately 3–7% CALLA + and/or B1 + cells in fetal livers of 11–26 weeks of gestation. The highest

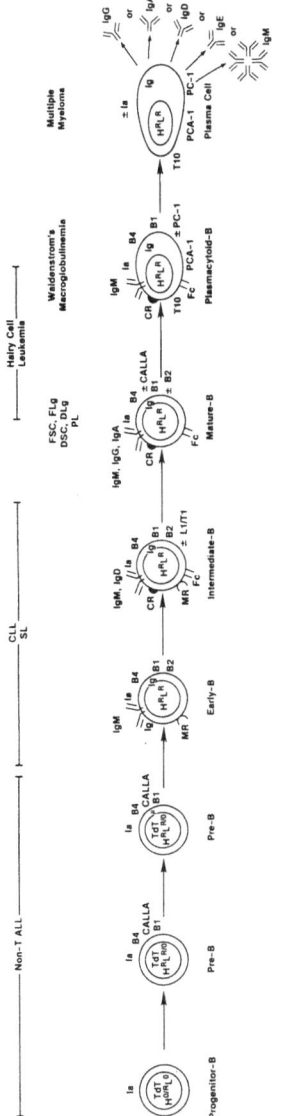

Figure 1.

48

Table 1. Reactivity of monoclonal anti-B-cell antibodies in fetal liver

Antibody	Gestation Age (wk)			
	11–14	15–17	18–22	22–26
CALLA	3	4	4	6
B1	1	2	2	7
B2	1	1	1	1
BA-1	4	–	–	1
RFB-1	3	–	–	< 1
TdT	5	4	1	< 1

numbers of positive cells were found in fetal livers of 22–26 weeks. B2 + cells were less common, occurring at a frequency of approximately 1% from 11 to 26 weeks. Budger and colleagues studied BA-1 and RFB-1 expression on fetal liver cells of 12–21 weeks gestation [14]. BA-1 + cells constituted 3–5% of fetal liver cells of 13 weeks gestation but only 1% of more mature fetal livers. RFB-1 + cells occurred at a slightly lower frequency. Both the BA-1 + RFB-1 + and BA-1 − RFB-1 + phenotypes were observed; many of the BA-1 + and/or RFB-1 + cells were also CALLA +. These investigators studied the relationship between TdT activity and surface antigens. TdT + was identified in 4–6% of early fetal liver cells and in 1% of more mature fetal liver cells. In 13 week fetal livers, 80% of TdT + cells were BA-1 + and RFB-1 +; the remaining 20% were BA-1 −, RFB-1 +. BA-1 + cells were more frequent than TdT + cells and were sIgM + suggesting that they were more mature B-cells. RFB-1 + cells also occurred more frequently than TdT + cells. These cells were sIgM − and were probably immature hematopoietic cells rather than lymphoid cells. Additional studies have also been performed using OKB1, 2, 4 and 7 monoclonal antibodies [16]. In most instances, fetal liver cells were OKB2 + but unreactive with other OKB antibodies.

When multiple B-cell specifications are studied simultaneously, it appears that most immature B cells are TdT +, B1 −, RFB-1 −, and Cμ −. These cells are probably progenitors of B1 + fetal liver cells, most of which are also RFB1 +, CALLA +, and OKB2 +. Approximately 15% of these cells contain Cμ and are probably best regarded as pre-B cells. Pre-B cells also express HLA-D/DR, β_2-microglobulin, and HLA-heavy chain but lack sIgM and TdT. As these cells mature to B cells they acquire sIgM, and possibly sIgD, and lose reactivity with RFB-1, CALLA, and OKB2; B1 and HLA reactivity is retained.

In summary, detailed analyses of human fetal liver B-lymphocytes using monoclonal antibodies are consistent with studies in other mammals. These indicate an orderly progression from hematopoietic stem cell progenitors to pre-B cells to B-cells and ultimately to mature B-lymphocytes and plasma cells. Most fetal liver cells are pre-B but several intermediate cell types are identified.

Functional studies of B- and T-lymphocytes in human and murine fetal liver cells have also been reported [2, 5, 6, 17, 18]. Transplantation results in a variable reconstitution of the B-lymphocyte axis in irradiated, fetal liver reconstituted mice [19–23]. Reconstitution is more complete in recipients of syngeneic transplants. Allograft recipients have less complete recovery of B-cell function [19, 24, 25]. These mice have decreased to low-normal levels of circulating Ig; antibody responses are present but decreased and IgM to IgG switching is impaired or absent. Analysis of fetal liver transplants in man, predominantly in patients with severe combined immune deficiency (SCID), indicate a low rate of permanent B-cell engraftment [26, 27]. This is probably related to the persistence of endogenous B-cells in these individuals. In dogs, we observed consistent B-cell engraftment with functional Ig and antibody responses after 6 months to 1 year [28]. Similar data by Prummer and coworkers have been reported [29]. In contrast to patients with SCID, these dogs are irradiated and achieve both lymphoid and hematopoietic engraftment. It is therefore conceivable that the functional B-cells in these animals arise from relatively uncommitted hematopoietic stem cells or B-cell progenitors rather than from pre-B or B-lymphocytes present in fetal liver. Irradiation of the recipient may also be a factor by providing 'space' in the lymphoid compartment for B-cell engraftment. Alternatively, the unirradiated recipient may have cells or factors which inhibit engraftment of immature B-cells.

In vitro studies of B-cells derived from fetal liver indicate the presence of functional B-cells responsive to polyclonal mitogens such as pokeweed mitogen (PWM). Specific antibody responses to sheep red blood cells following in vivo immunization of mice indicate present but decreased anti-SRBC plaque-forming cells (PFC). Normal responses to dextran and lipopolysaccharide have been reported in mice [23]. Detailed studies using other antigens in vivo or in vitro have not been reported nor have in vitro studies in man.

Hannam-Harris and Smith analyzed Ig synthesis by human fetal liver cells by biosynthetic labeling [30]. Fetal liver cells synthesized and secreted free Ig light chain; some cells also secreted free heavy chain. This imbalance in Ig light chain synthesis is thought to be typical of immature B cells (pre-B) and is also found in B-cells from patients with chronic lymphocytic leukemia. The specificity of antibodies produced in cultures of fetal liver cells is unknown in most instances. Some data indicate the presence of anti-idiotype antibodies specific for autoantigens. Interestingly, several dogs transplanted with fetal liver cells have developed autoantibodies and occasionally autoimmune diseases such as myasthenia gravis or idiopathic thrombocytopenic purpura (ITP) [31]. The frequency of autoimmune diseases appears increased compared to canine recipients of bone marrow transplants; this may be related to the relative immaturity of B-cells in fetal liver.

In summary, fetal liver is the major site of B-lymphocyte development in the human fetus. Mature B-cells that can synthesize Ig and probably antibody arise from B-cell progenitors. B-lymphocytes, derived from fetal liver stem cells or their progeny, are capable of restoring B-cell immunity in mice and dogs; data in man are less convincing but this may be related to factors other than the immune competence of the stem cells transplanted.

T-lymphocyte development

In contrast to B-lymphocyte development which occurs primarily in the fetal liver, T-lymphocyte development occurs primarily in the thymus. Nevertheless, most if not all T-cells arise from fetal liver progenitors. In mice, rats, dogs, minipigs, sheep, horses, monkeys and man, transplantation of fetal liver cells alone or in combination with thymus cells results in restoration of T-cell immunity [2, 3, 23–29, 31–48]. T-cell recovery is impaired if the recipient is thymectomized suggesting that most of the fetal liver cells responsible for T-cell reconstitution are pre-thymic [23].

Attempts to demonstrate mature T-lymphocytes in human fetal liver have been unsuccessful [5, 6, 17, 18, 49]. E-rosette forming cells, T-cells capable of binding sheep red blood cells, are present at < 1% frequency. Recent studies have used monoclonal anti-T cell antibodies including T1, 3, 4, 6, and 5/8, Leu 1,2 and 3, and T101 [13, 15]. In all instances, < 2% of positive cells are found suggesting the absence of mature T-cells in fetal liver.

Functional analyses of T-cells in human fetal liver include studies of reactivity to alloantigens in mixed leukocyte culture (MLC), and to mitogens including phytohemagglutinin A (PHA) and concanavalin A (conA). We and others studied MLC reactivity of fetal liver cells [5, 17, 49–52]. Most studies indicate that these cells are unreactive or only slightly reactive in MLC. Studies which suggested strong MLC reactivity, in all likelihood measured the response of myeloid rather than lymphoid cells. There have been several studies of mitogen-induced reactivity of fetal liver cells [17, 18, 49–54]. In most instances only weak reactivity to PHA and no response to conA was detected. This pattern of reactivity is consistent with other species where development of PHA reactivity preceeds conA reactivity.

In sheep fetal liver cells appear to be reactive in MLC. Interestingly and in contrast to mature T-cells, cytotoxic lymphocytes could not be demonstrated [55]. Irradiated dogs reconstituted with fetal liver cells recovered mitogen responsiveness within 3 months; MLC reactivity recovered less rapidly but relatively few animals have been studied [28, 29, 32, 33]. Data in dogs from ourselves and Prummer and coworkers suggest that B-cell recovery preceeds T-cell recovery. This was unanticipated since, in man, T-cell rather than B-cell engraftment is more easily achieved [27, 40, 71]. These differences may be species specific or may be related to either DLA-matching between donor and recipient or to the fact that recipients were irradiated and therefore achieved complete hematopoietic grafts rather than only lymphoid grafts. Several investigators have evaluated T-cell content of human fetal livers by histochemical techniques such as reactivity with acid alpha-naphthyl acetate esterase (ANAE). ANAE reactive cells were not detected in fetal livers < 14 weeks; 1–3% were detectable thereafter increasing to 5–7% by 24 weeks and then declined [53]. These data are in agreement with studies using monoclonal antibodies.

Despite the relative absence of mature T-cells in fetal liver, T-cell progenitors are clearly present. We studied the colony forming cells (CFU-TL) in semi-solid agar in 15 fetal livers of 10 to 24 weeks gestation [28, 49]. CFU-TL were present at a frequency similar to that observed in adult bone marrow. In these instances there was no correlation between CFU-TL and the presence of E-rosette forming cells or reactivity to PHA. These data suggest that the CFU-TL, under these circumstances, are indicative of T-cell progenitors rather than mature T-cells. Cells recovered from CFU-TL colonies had the phenotype of mature T-cells and were alloantigen and mitogen reactive. Similarly Pyke and Gelfand and Lowenberg have reported T-cell progenitors in human fetal liver [56, 70].

Rabinowich and coworkers have studied T-cell progenitors in murine fetal liver [23]. They reported that irradiated mice reconstituted with fetal liver cells were similar to bone marrow chimeras in their ability to reject thyroid allografts, and in their reactivity to alloantigens, PHA and conA. In general these responses recovered less rapidly following fetal liver than bone marrow transplantation and were markedly impaired or absent in thymectomized recipients. Interestingly, these investigators also reported that B-cell responses recovered more rapidly than T-cell responses similar to the aforementioned results in dogs and in contrast to results in patients with SCID receiving fetal liver grafts.

Natural killer cells

Recently, there has been interest in natural killer (NK) cells which react with selected target cells without prior sensitization [57]. The origin of NK cells is controversial and it is uncertain whether they are T-cells, or monocyte/macrophages, or both. NK cells appear to be distinct from K cells which mediate antibody dependent cellular cytotoxicity (ADCC). NK cells are present in murine fetal liver cells [58, 59]. Toivanen and coworkers detected NK activity in most human fetal livers of 9–23 weeks gestation [53]. This activity could be increased by incubation with interferon similar to NK cells from other sources.

Regulation of immunity by fetal liver cells

There are considerable data indicating that transplantation of fetal liver cells is associated with a lower incidence and severity of graft-versus-host disease (GvHD) in animal models and man [2, 3]. The most obvious explanation of decreased GvHD is the relative immune incompetence of fetal liver cells. This may arise from several factors: (1) absent or infrequent mature T-lymphocytes; (2) education of donor derived T-cell progenitors in the recipient thymus; or (3) the relative ease of tolerization of clonal deletion of alloantigen reactive fetal liver cells.

Another possible explanation of the decreased immune reactivity of fetal liver cells is their unique immunoregulatory features. Several investigators have reported suppressor T-cells in murine fetal liver [60–64]. Recently, Muraoka and Miller demonstrated that murine fetal liver cells or cells from fetal liver CFU-TL colonies specifically suppress reactivity of allogeneic lymphocytes to self [65]. This anti-self suppressor effect is mediated by fetal liver derived cells and appears to act by preventing differentiation of cytotoxic-T-cell precursors into cytotoxic effector cells. The suppressor cells are termed 'veto' cells to distinguish them from other types of suppressor cells. These 'veto' cells appear to be non-T, non-B cells and are relatively radioresistant. Sula and Nouza reported a similar observation in mice whereby addition of fetal liver cells syngeneic to the recipient decreased regional GvHD in irradiated recipients [66].

In summary it appears that fetal liver contains cell(s) capable of regulating reactivity of immune competent cells either present in the fetal liver or allogeneic to the fetal liver cells. This regulatory aspect of fetal liver immune development may be important in the normal regulation of anti-self immunity as well as in the setting of fetal liver transplantation. In the latter, 'veto' cells would tend to suppress the ability of the recipient to reject the graft.

Interactions of fetal liver and T-cells

Interesting observations have been made regarding the interaction of fetal liver cells with other immune cells, particularly thymocytes. Bortin and coworkers reported that addition of syngeneic thymocytes increased the likelihood of successful fetal liver transplantation in mice [63, 67]. Relatively small numbers of thymocytes were effective. These authors suggested that this activity was mediated by a soluble factor since thymi transplanted within millipore filters had the same activity as intact thymocytes.

The precise mechanism by which this effect occurs is unknown. These investigators reported successful engraftment of an irradiated dog following multiple fetal liver and thymus grafts [68]. It is not possible to conclude whether engraftment was a consequence of the combined use of fetal liver and thymus or would have been achieved with fetal liver cells alone. Perryman has reported similar data in horses [45]. Touraine and coworkers and others have reported results of combined fetal liver and thymus transplants in man [41, 69]; again critical analyses are not possible, since the small number of patients did not permit definite conclusions on the role of the added thymus.

In summary, there are reasonably convincing data in rodents that thymocytes increase the probability of successful engraftment of fetal liver cells; data in other species are less certain. This effect may not require intact cells and therefore need not necessarily increase the risk of GvHD. Controlled trials of this approach in man are needed.

Conclusion

Human fetal liver contains progenitors of both B- and T-cells capable of restoring humoral and cellular immunity in irradiated, fetal liver reconstituted recipients. The fetal liver is the major site of B-cell development in man. Although maturation of T-cells occurs primarily in the thymus, the fetal liver contains T-cell progenitors and is critical to T-cell development. Other immune functions of fetal liver cells, such as NK activity, are probably also present but have not been studied in detail. Fetal liver cells appear to have relatively unique self-regulatory functions which may play in important role in the maintenance of tolerance to self and in the prevention of graft-rejection and GvHD following fetal liver transplantation. Transplantation of fetal liver cells and thymocytes appears to be more effective than fetal liver cells alone in rodents; controlled trials in large animals and man are needed. Recent studies in dogs support that it is possible to achieve long-term survival and immune reconstitution following transplantation of a single, DLA matched fetal liver. Based on these data it may be possible to undertake comparable transplants in man.

References

1. Keleman E, Calvo W, Fliedner TM: Atlas of Human Hematopoietic Development. Springer-Verlag, Berlin, 1979
2. Lowenberg B: Fetal liver transplantation. Radiobiological Institute of the Organization for Health Research TNO, Rijswijk, the Netherlands, 1975
3. Lucarelli G, Andreani M, Agostinelli F: Fetal liver transplantation in rats. In: Lucarelli G, Fliedner TM, Gale RP (eds) Fetal Liver Transplantation: Current Concepts and Future Directions. Excerpta Medica, Amsterdam, 1980, pp 175

4. Fliedner TM, Calvo W: Current concepts and future directions of fetal liver transplantation. In: Lucarelli G, Fliedner TM, Gale RP (eds) Fetal Liver Transplantation. Excerpta Medica, Amsterdam. 1980, pp 305
5. Prindull G: Maturation of cellular and humoral immunity during human embryonic development. Acta Pediatr Scand 63: 607, 1974
6. Stites DP, Caldwell J, Carr MC, Fudenberg HH: Ontogeny of immunity in humans. Clin Immunol Immunopath 4: 519, 1975
7. Gathings WE, Kubogawa H, Cooper MD: A distinctive pattern of B-cell immaturity in perinatal humans. Immunol Rev 57: 107–28, 1981
8. Calvert JE, Maruyama S, Tedder TF, Webb CF, Cooper MD: Cellular events in the differentiation of antibody secreting cells. Sem Hematol 21: 226, 1984
9. LeDouarin NM, Houssaint E, Joterean FV, Belo M: Origin of hematopoietic stem cells in the embryonic bursa of Fabricius and bone marrow studied through inter-specific chimeras. Proc Natl Acad Sci USA 72: 2701, 1975
10. Owen JJ, Weight DE, Habu S, Raff MC, Cooper MD: Studies on the generation of B-lymphocytes in fetal liver and bone marrow. J Immunol 118: 2067, 1977
11. Kamps WA, Cooper MD: Microenvironmental studies of pre-B and B-cell development in human and mouse fetuses. J Immunol 129: 526, 1982
12. Kincade PW, Phillips RA: B lymphocyte development. Fed Proceed 44: 2874, 1985
13. Rosenthal P, Rimm IJ, Umiel T et al.: Ontogeny of human hematopoietic cells: Analysis using monoclonal antibodies. J Immunol 131: 232, 1983
14. Budger MP, Janossy G, Bollum FJ, Burford GD, Hoffbrand AV: The ontogeny of terminal deoxynucleotidyl transferase positive cells in the human fetus. Blood 61: 1125, 1983
15. De Biagi, Andreani M, Centis F: Immune characterization of human fetal tissues with monoclonal antibodies. In: Gale RP, Touraine J-L, Lucarelli G (eds) Fetal Liver Transplantation. AR Liss, New York, 1985, pp 89
16. Knowles DM, II, Tolidjian B, Marboe CC et al.: Distribution of antigens defined by OKB monoclonal antibodies on benign and malignant lymphoid cells and on nonlymphoid tissue. Blood 63: 886–896, 1984
17. Mukopadhyay N, Fernbach DJ, Mumford DM, South MA: T- and B-cells and immune competence in human fetal liver cells. Clin Immunol Immunopath 10: 59, 1978
18. Delfini C, Izzi T, Porcellini A, Lucarelli G: Immunologic features of human fetal liver, spleen and thymus of various gestational ages. In: Lucarelli G, Fliedner TM, Gale RP (eds) Fetal Liver Transplantation: Current Concepts, Future Directions. Excerpta Medica, Amsterdam, 1980, pp 126
19. Doria G, Goodman JW, Gengozian N, Congdon CC: Immunologic study of antibody-forming cells in mouse radiation chimeras. J Immunol 88: 20, 1962
20. Tyan ML, Cole LJ, Herzenberg LA: Fetal Liver: A source of immunoglobulin producing cells in the mouse. Proc Soc Exp Biol Med 124: 161, 1967
21. Umiel T, Globerson A: Analysis of lymphoid cell types developing in the mouse fetal liver. Differentiation 2: 169, 1974
22. Rosenberg YJ, Cunningham AJ: Ontogeny of the antibody-forming cell line in mice. III The generation of mature antisheep red blood cell-specific B-cells is antigen dependent. Eur J Immunol 7: 257, 1977
23. Rabinowich H, Umiel T, Globerson A: T-cell progenitors in the mouse fetal liver. Transplantation 35: 40, 1983
24. Gengozian N, Rabette B, Congdon CC: Abnormal immune mechanism in allogeneic radiation chimeras. Science 149: 645, 1965
25. Gengozian N, Congdon CC: Immunologic memory in radiation chimeras. Transplantation 16: 32, 1973
26. O'Reilly RJ, Pahwa R, Sorrell M, et al.: Transplantation of fetal liver and thymus in patients with severe combined immunodeficiencies. In: Doria G, Eshkol A (eds) The Immune System: Functions and Therapy of Dysfunctions. Academic Press, 1978, pp 241
27. Gale RP: Immune development in human fetal liver. In: Gale RP, Touraine J-L, Lucarelli G (eds) Fetal Liver Transplantation. AR Liss, New York, 1985, pp 73
28. Champlin RE, Cain G, Stitzel K, Gale RP: Fetal liver cell transplantation in dogs: Results with DLA-compatible and incompatible grafts. In: Gale RP, Touraine J-L, Lucarelli G (eds) Fetal Liver Transplantation. AR Liss, New York, 1985, pp 195

29. Prummer O, Calvo W, Werner C, Corbonell F, Fliedner TM: Hemopoiesis and immune function in dogs following fetal liver transplantation. In: Gale RP, Touraine J-L, Lucarelli G (eds) Fetal Liver Transplantation. AR Liss, New York, 1985, pp 175

30. Hannam-Harris AC, Smith JL: Free immunoglobulin light chain synthesis by human fetal liver and cord blood lymphocytes. Immunol 43: 417, 1981

31. Cain GR, Cardinett III GN, Cuddon PC, Gale RP, Champlin RE: Myasthenia gravis and polymyositis in a dog following fetal hematopietic cell transplantation. Transplantation, in press.

32. Prummer O, Werner C, Raghavachar A, Nothdurft W, Calvo W, Steinbach K-H, Fliedner TM: Fetal liver transplantation in the dog. Transplantation 40: 498, 1985

33. Prummer O, Raghavachar A, Werner C et al.: Fetal liver transplantation in the dog: I. Restoration of hempoiesis with cryo-preserved fetal liver cells from DLA-identical siblings. Transplantation 39: 349, 1985

34. Andreani M, De Biagi M, Centis F, Manna M et al.: Fetal liver transplantation in the mini-pig. In: Gale RP, Touraine J-L, Lucarelli G (eds) Fetal Liver Transplantation. AR Liss, New York, 1985, pp 205

35. Bunch C, Wood WG, Kelly SJ: Fetal hematopoietic-cell transplantation in sheep: An approach to the cellular control of hemoglobin switching. In: Gale RP, Touraine J-L, Lucarelli G (eds) Fetal Liver Transplantation. AR Liss, New York, 1985, pp 219

36. Kochupillai V, Sharma S, Francis S et al.: Bone marrow reconstitution following human fetal liver infusion (FLI) in sixteen severe aplastic anemia patients. In: Gale RP, Touraine J-L, Lucarelli G (eds) Fetal Liver Transplantation. AR Liss, New York, 1985, pp 237

37. Kochupillai V, Sharma S, Francis S et al.: Fetal liver infusion: An adjuvant in the theory of acute myeloid leukemia (AML). In: Gale RP, Touraine J-L, Lucarelli G (eds) Fetal Liver Transplantation. AR Liss, New York, 1985, pp 267

38. Izzi T, Polchi P, Galimberti M et al.: Fetal Liver Transplantation in aplastic anemia and acute leukemia. In: Gale RP, Touraine J-L, Lucarelli G (eds) Fetal Liver Transplantation. AR Liss, New York, 1985, pp 237

39. Meng P-L, Fei R-G, Gu D-W, Yie W-Z et al.: Allogenic fetal liver transplantation in acute leukemia. In: Gale RP, Touraine J-L, Lucarelli G (eds) Fetal Liver Transplantation. AR Liss, New York, 1985, pp 281

40. Gale RP: Fetal liver transplantation in man. In: Lucarelli G, Fliedner TM, Gale RP (eds) Fetal Liver Transplantation: Current Concepts and Future Directions. Excerpta Medica, Amsterdam, 1980, pp 268

41. Touraine J-L: Transplantation of both fetal liver and thymus in severe combined immunodeficiencies: Interaction between donor and recipient cells. In: Lucarelli G, Fliedner TM, Gale RP (eds) Fetal Liver Transplantation: Current Concepts and Future Directions. Excerpta Medica, Amsterdam, 1980, pp 276

42. Bortin MM, Rimm AA, Saltzstein EC: Survival and immune competence of murine radiation chimeras. Fed Proc 30: 652, 1971

43. Bortin MM, Rimm AA, Saltzstein EC: Graft-versus-host inhibition. IV. Production of allogeneic radiation chimeras using incubated spleen and liver cell mixtures. J Immunol 107: 1063, 1971

44. van Putten LM, van Bekkum DW, deVries MJ: Transplantation of fetal hematopoietic cells in irradiated rhesus monkeys. In: Radiation and the Control of the Immune Response. Internatl Atomic Energy Comm, Vienna, 1968, p 41

45. Perryman LE: Use of fetal tissue for immune reconstitution in horses with severe combined immunodeficiency. In: Lucarelli G, Fliedner TM, Gale RP (eds) Fetal Liver Transplantation: Current Concepts and Future Directions. Excerpta Medica, Amsterdam, 1980, pp 183

46. Stutman O: Intrathymic and extrathymic T-cell maturation. Immunol Rev 42: 138, 1978

47. Umiel T, Globerson A, Auerbach R: Role of the thymus in the development of immunocompetence of embryonic liver cells in vitro. Proc Soc Exp Biol Med 129: 598, 1968

48. Hunt SV, Fowler MH: A repopulation assay for B and T lymphocyte stem cells employing radiation chimeras. Cell Tissue Kinetics 14: 445, 1981

49. Champlin RE, Niskanen E, Gale RP: Hematopoiesis and immunereactivity of human fetal liver cells. In: Lucarelli G, Fliedner TM, Gale RP (eds) Fetal Liver Transplantation. Excerpta Medica, Amsterdam, 1980, pp 117

50. August CS, Berkel AJ, Driscoll S, Marler E: Onset of lymphocyte function in the developing human fetus. Pediatr Res 5: 5329, 1971
51. Carr MC, Stites DP, Fudenberg HH: Dissociation of response to phytohemaglutinin and adult allogeneic lymphocytes in human foetal tissues. Nature New Biol 241: 279, 1973
52. Stites DP, Carr MC, Fudenberg HH: Ontogeny of cellular immunity in the human fetus. Cell Immunol 11: 257, 1974
53. Toivanen P, Uksila J, Leino A, Lassila O, Hirvonen T, Ruuskanen O: Development of mitogen responding T-cells and natural killer cells in the human fetus. Immunol Rev 57: 89–105, 1981
54. Sirianni MC, Fiorilli M, Casadei AM, Auiti F: Response to B- and T-cell mitogens and surface markers in human fetal lymphoid tissues. Thymus 1: 257, 1980
55. Granberg C, Hirvonen T: Cell-mediated lympholysis by fetal and neonatal lymphocytes in sheep and man. Cell Immunol 51: 13, 1980
56. Pyke KW, Gelfand EW: Detection of T precursor cells in human bone marrow and foetal liver. Differentiation 5: 189–191, 1976
57. Herberman RB, Ortaldo JR: Natural killer cells: Their role in defenses against disease. Science 214: 24, 1981
58. Koo GC, Peppard JR, Hatzfeld A: Ontogeny of NK-1 + natural killer cells. 1. Proportion of NK-1 + cells in fetal, baby and old mice. J Immunol 129: 867, 1982
59. Haller O, Kiessling R, Orn A, Wigzell H: Generation of natural killer cells: an autonomous function of the bone marrow. J Exp Med 145: 1411, 1977
60. Globerson A, Zinkernagel RM, Umiel T: Immunosuppression by embryonic liver cells. Transplantation 20: 480, 1975
61. Globerson A, Umiel T: Ontogeny of suppressor cells. II. Supression of graft-versus-host disease and mixed leukocyte cultures by embryonic cells. Transplantation 26: 438, 1978
62. Umiel T: Development of specific suppressor cells of embryonic or neonatal fetal liver origin and their possible role in immunological tolerance. In: Solomon JB, Horton JD (eds). Op cit p 323, 1977
63. Bortin MM, Rimm AA, Saltzstein EC: Graft-versus-host inhibition. I. Incubated parental strain spleen and liver cells administered to F_1 mice. J Immunol 102: 1042, 1969
64. Bortin MM, Saltzstein EC: Graft-versus-host inhibition. Fetal liver and thymus cells to minimize secondary disease. Science 164: 316, 1969
65. Muraoka S, Miller RG: Cells in murine fetal liver and in lymphoid colonies grown from fetal liver can suppress generation of cytotoxic T-lymphocytes directed against their self antigen. J Immunol 131: 45, 1983
66. Sula K, Nouza K: Immunogenetic requirements for regulatory effects of fetal cells. In: Hraba T, Hasek M (eds) Cellular and Molecular Mechanisms of Immunologic Tolerance. Marcel Dekker, New York, 1981, p 161
67. Bortin MM, Rimm AA, Saltzstein EC: Potentiating effect of fetal thymus on fetal liver cells for the promotion of recovery from the radiation injury in murine allogeneic radiation chimeras or a little bit of thymus goes a long, long way. Birth Defects: Original Article Series, 11: 544, 1975
68. Saltzstein EC, Bortin MM, Rimm AA, Hussey JL: Long lived canine allogeneic radiation chimera produced with combined fetal liver and thymus cells. Transplantation 18: 461, 1974
69. Touraine J-L, Roncarolo MG, Marseglia GL et al: Fetal liver transplantation in immunodeficiencies and inborn errors of metabolism. In: Gale RP, Touraine J-L, Lucarelli G (eds) Fetal Liver Transplantation. AR Liss, New York, 1985, pp 299
70. Lowenberg B: Lymphocyte maturation and graft-versus-host disease following fetal liver transplantation. In: Lucarelli G, Fliedner TM, Gale RP (eds) Fetal Liver Transplantation. Excerpta Medica, Amsterdam, 1980, pp 198
71. O'Reilly RS, Kirkpatrick D, Kapoor N et al.: A comparative review of the results of transplants of fully allogeneic fetal liver and HLA-haplotype mismatched, T-cell depleted marrow in the treatment of severe combined immunodeficiency. In: Gale RP, Touraine J-L, Lucarelli G (eds) Fetal Liver Transplantation. AR Liss, New York, 1985, pp 327

Thymus 10:57–73 (1987)

Ontogeny of T lymphocyte differentiation in the human fetus: Acquisition of phenotype and functions

C. ROYO, J.-L. TOURAINE[1] and O. DE BOUTEILLER

Transplantation and Immunobiology Unit, Pavillon P, Hôpital Edouard Herriot, F-69437 Lyon Cédex 08, France

(*Accepted 15 May 1987*)

Key words: human fetus, lymphoid organs, T lymphocytes, ontogeny

Summary. Phenotype and functions of cells of the T lymphocyte lineage from fetal liver, thymus, spleen and bone marrow were investigated at various ages. T lymphocyte differentiation was shown to be initiated in the thymus after the 7th week of gestation. In this organ, a large number of cells with a phenotype comparable to that of children thymocytes and with a high proliferative response to phytomitogens was observed at the 14th week. The fetal liver and bone marrow never contained many T-cells and the liver was shown to be virtually devoid of any of these cells before the 13th week. Fetal spleen contained appreciable amounts of T-cells after the 13th week. Helper and suppressor activities of fetal thymocytes and splenocytes were acquired between the 12th and the 16th week, but they were never as complete nor as potent as those of adult lymphocytes. HLA antigens were detected in very low amount in lymphocytes from the various organs at the beginning of the second trimester and their expression was significantly enhanced by in vitro incubation with α-interferon (α-IFN), a procedure that permits easier HLA typing of fetal cells.

Introduction

The developing field of fetal liver and thymus transplantation requires basic knowledge on ontogeny of lymphopoiesis and haematopoiesis. It is of special importance to characterize the various stages of development of T lymphocytes from stem cells and, in each organ, to identify the period of appearance of T-cells able to induce graft-versus-host disease (GvHD). Initial studies had shown that T-cell development was both quantitatively and qualitatively important during the second trimester of gestation [14, 4]. The interpretation of the mixed leucocyte reactivities was uncertain since non T-cells could play a part in such responses [14].

We have undertaken a systematic analysis of T-cell markers, mitogen responses, suppressor and helper activities, in fetal lymphoid organs between the 7th and 25th week of gestation. This investigation has confirmed that fetal liver is a source of stem cells naturally devoid of a significant population of T lymphocytes. The thymus is mostly an epithelial organ

---

[1] Author for correspondence.

until the 8th week, and it contains a large number of thymocytes with some functional activities from the 13th week onwards.

The findings in human fetuses can be used as a rationale for selecting fetal organs of appropriate ages for transplantation purposes, as well as for development of cell lines of fetal origin. They also provide informations on the natural sequences of events on the process of T-cell differentiation. Precise knowledge on these stages has proven useful for a careful monitoring of immunological reconstitution following fetal liver transplants, especially in patients with severe combined immunodeficiency [19].

Materials and methods

Tissue samples

Most human fetuses were obtained from therapeutic, prostaglandin-induced abortions. A few additional fetuses came from extra-uterine pregnancies or from hysterotomies when the mother's condition required surgery. In all instances, the rules defined by the Ethical Committee of Claude Bernard University were carefully followed.

Fetal tissues were processed within 1 to 8 hours after delivery. The post-fecundation (PF) age was calculated from the date of the last menstruation minus 2 weeks, and from the foot length, according to Streeter's data [15]. It ranged from 7 to 25 weeks.

Cell preparation

Fetal cell suspensions were prepared from the thymus, the liver, the spleen and the bone marrow. The thymus, liver and spleen were gently homogenized in RPMI-1640 culture medium using a tissue grinder. Bone marrow cells were obtained by flushing marrow plugs from femurs with RPMI-1640 medium. The cell suspensions were washed once. The cell viability was determined by the Trypan Blue exclusion method and all samples with a viability below 60% were discarded. Liver, spleen and bone marrow samples were then enriched in mononuclear cells by centrifugation over a Ficoll-Hypaque gradient [3]. The cell viability was always higher than 90% after Ficoll-Hypaque separation.

Monoclonal antibodies

OKT3, OKT4, OKT6, OKT8 and OKT11 mouse monoclonal antibodies (MoAb), specific for T-cell differentiation antigens, were purchased from Ortho Pharmaceutical Corporation (Raritan, NJ). OKT9, OKT10 and OKIa1 MoAb were also obtained from Ortho Pharmaceuticals Corporation. The anti-human β2-microglobulin (B2-m) and Leu-7 MoAb, as well as phycoerythrin-labeled-Leu 3a and -Leu 2a MoAb were supplied by Becton Dickinson Company (Mountain View, CA).

Indirect immunofluorescence assay

The appropriate amount of each MoAb (5 μl) was added to 10^6 cells. After a 30 min incubation period at 4 °C, cells were washed in PBS supplemented with 2% bovine serum albumin (BSA) and 0.1% sodium azide (NaN$_3$). The supernatants were removed and 20 μl of 1:5 dilution of fluorescein-labeled goat anti-mouse (IgG + IgM + IgA) antiserum (Coultronics, Hialeah, FL) were added. After 30 min at 4 °C, the cells were washed twice and the supernatants removed. Stained cells were then resuspended at a concentration of 2 × 10^6 cells per ml in PBS with 0.1% NaN$_3$. They were then processed for flow cytometry analysis (Ortho H50, Ortho Instruments, Westword, MA). 10 000 cells per sample were analyzed for surface antigens. Forward angle scatter was used to gate lymphocyte population, and 90 ° light scatter to eliminate residual erythrocytes and dead cells. Histograms of cell numbers plotted against fluorescence intensity were recorded. The percentage of positive cells in each sample was calculated after subtraction of the reactivity of cells incubated with fluorescein-labeled anti-mouse immunoglobulin serum only.

Induction assay with interferon

Recombinant α2-IFN (specific activity: 5 × 10^8 IU/mg protein) was kindly provided by Dr A. Waitz (DNAX, Palo Alto, CA).

Mononuclear cells from the thymus, the liver and the spleen of 7–23 week-old fetuses were incubated with α2-IFN (30 IU/ml) at a concentration of 10^6 cells per ml in RPMI-1640 culture medium complemented with L-glutamin (2 mM/l), penicillin (100 U/ml), streptomycin (50 μg/ml) (Biomérieux, Marcy l'Etoile, France) and inactivated human AB serum (10%). Following a 24 hr incubation period at 37 °C in 5% CO$_2$-95% air, the cells were harvested and washed. They were then incubated with OKT10, OKT3, OKT4, OKT6, OKT8, OKT11 and anti-β2-m monoclonal antibodies. Fluorescein-labeled anti-mouse immunoglobulin was added as described above. Control samples were incubated in the same medium, but in the absence of α2-IFN, then labeled using the same monoclonal antibodies.

Mitogen responsiveness

Mononuclear cells from fetal thymus, spleen and liver were resuspended at a concentration of 10^6 cells per ml in RPMI-1640 culture medium supplemented with L-glutamin, antibiotics and AB serum. 2 × 10^5 cells were introduced in each well of a microplate. Phytohemagglutinin (PHA, Wellcome Laboratories, Dartford, England), Concanavalin A (ConA, Sigma, St Louis, MO) or Pokeweed Mitogen (PWM, Gibco, Grand Island, NY) were added at final dilutions of respectively 1/400, 100 μg/ml and 1/60. Cells were incubated 3 days in 5% CO$_2$-95% air. The cell proliferation over the last 18 hrs of the 3 day culture was determined by the incorporation of 3H-Thymidine (CEA, Saclay, France) measured in a liquid scintillation counter. Results were expressed in desintegrations per minute (dpm, mean ± S.D.).

Suppressor activity

The suppressor activity of the various cell suspensions from fetal thymus and spleen, at ages of 12–22 weeks, was determined following ConA activation, as previously described for peripheral blood lymphocytes (PBL) of adult origin [18].

Helper activity

Mononuclear cells from 12 to 23 week-old thymuses and spleens were cultured at a concentration of 10^6 cells per ml in RPMI-1640 culture medium supplemented with L-glutamin, penicillin, streptomycin and 10% inactivated fetal calf serum, in the presence of PWM (1/400) for 7 days at 37 °C in 5% CO_2-95% air. The percentage of cells with intracytoplasmic immunoglobulin (IGM + IgG + IgA) was determined using an immunofluorescence method adapted to intracellular labeling [13].

To analyze the capacity of fetal B-cells to differentiate into plasmacytoid cells and the capacity of fetal T-cells to help B-cell differentiation, fetal spleen cells were separated into T- and B-cells (T-cells were obtained by filtration through a nylon wool column and B-cells by elimination of AET-rosettes). Fetal T-cells were then incubated with B-cells from adult PBL in the presence of PWM; vice versa fetal B-cells were incubated with adult T-cells and PWM.

Results and discussion

Surface markers of T-cell differentiation

At all fetal ages analyzed, less than 2% of cells from the fetal liver and less than 10% of the cells from the fetal bone marrow expressed the T-cell differentiation antigens, i.e. T3, T4, T6, T8 and T11 (Tables 1 and 2). At the same ontogenetic stages, the majority of thymocytes expressed these antigens, with a simultaneous expression of T4, T8 and T6 antigens (Table 3 and Figure 1). Lymphocytes were detected in appreciable number in the spleen from the 12th week. At this period and thereafter, only a low percentage of cells expressed simultaneous T4 and T8 antigens while the majority of splenocytes expressed either T4 or T8 antigens, and have acquired the T3 antigen expression (Table 4).

T-cell specific antigens were therefore rapidly expressed by lymphoid cells after they had colonized the thymus. Following their intra-thymic differentiation, cells migrated to peripheral lymphoid organs, with only few T-cells returning to the bone marrow and even less T-cells returning to the fetal liver. These results are in agreement with the schemes of

Table 1. Surface markers expressed by fetal liver mononuclear cells.

MoAb	Gestational age (weeks PF)						
	7	12	14	15	17	21	23
OKT11	< 0.5[a]	< 0.5	0.5	1.4	1	1.2	1.2
OKT3	0.5	0.5	0.5	1.0	1	< 0.5	< 0.5
OKT4	0.5	0.5	0.5	1.2	0.9	0.5	0.5
OKT8	0.5	0.5	0.5	1.1	1.0	0.7	1.7
OKT6	N.D.	< 0.5	< 0.5	1.0	0.8	0.5	0.8
OKT9	20.0	24.0	40.0	37.0	40.0	52.0	37.0
OKT10	5.0	10.0	4.0	11.0	37.0	62.0	76.0
β2-m	4.0	14.0	10.0	19.0	26.0	35.0	46.0
OKIa1	3.0	11.0	7.0	11.0	17.0	35.0	47.0
Leu-7	< 0.1	< 0.1	< 0.1	< 0.1	< 0.1	< 0.1	< 0.1

[a]Percentage of positive cells as determined by flow cytometry analysis.

Table 2. Surface markers expressed by fetal bone marrow mononuclear cells.

MoAb	Gestational age (weeks PF)					
	14	15	16	20	21	23
OKT11	< 0.5[a]	< 0.5	< 0.5	< 0.5	< 0.5	< 1.0
OKT3	0.7	1.0	1.1	1.0	5.0	8.0
OKT4	< 0.5	1.1	1.1	1.0	1.5	3.8
OKT8	0.6	0.8	0.9	4.0	5.0	6.0
OKT6	< 0.5	< 0.5	< 0.5	< 0.5	0.8	1.1
OKT10	8.0	20.0	42.0	29.0	51.0	83.0
β2-m	10.0	19.0	26.0	40.0	46.0	52.0
OKIa1	11.0	15.0	15.0	41.0	36.0	46.0
Leu-7	< 0.1	< 0.1	< 0.1	< 0.1	< 0.1	< 0.1

[a]Percentage of positive cells as determined by flow cytometry analysis.

T-lymphocyte differentiation described by Reinherz et al. [11] and by Asma et al. [2].

Class I and class II HLA antigens were weakly expressed at the cell surface of lymphoid cells from fetal liver and bone marrow. Class II HLA antigens were virtually not detected on thymocytes at any fetal age, while class I HLA antigens were expressed, at a low density, by 90% of thymocytes from the 14th week onwards. In the spleen, these class I antigens were found on 83% of cells as a mean; class II antigens were detected on 38% of fetal spleen cells.

In all four organs, a large percentage of cells expressed the T10 antigens, which do not appear to be specific for a lymphocyte subpopulation but rather for some early stages of differentiation in several cell lineages [11, 7]. The T9 antigens were weakly expressed by fetal thymocytes, while these antigens were detected on a relatively large number of fetal liver and spleen cells.

A very low percentage (< 0.1%) of Leu-7-positive cells was consistently found in these fetal organs before the 24th. These results are comparable

Table 3. Surface markers expressed by fetal thymocytes.

MoAb	Gestational age (weeks PF)												
	7	8	9	13	14	15	16	17	18	20	21	23	25
OKT11	69[a]	58	76	73	89.5 ± 0.7	98	96	81	89.0 ± 0.3	94.0 ± 0.7	90.0 ± 0.7	91	94.0 ± 0.2
OKT3	13	17	18	34	51.5 ± 9.0	50	35	47	39.0 ± 0.7	48.0 ± 20.0	78.0 ± 29.0	39	70.0 ± 1.5
OKT4	28	60	36	80	69.5 ± 5.0	89	48	76	84.0 ± 4.0	88.0 ± 8.0	96.0 ± 2.0	58	93.0 ± 2.0
OKT8	31	58	45	58	77.5 ± 13.0	82	59	78	79.0 ± 6.5	86.5 ± 6.0	96.0 ± 1.5	65	92.0 ± 1.0
OKT6	N.D.	55	N.D.	72	75.5 ± 6.5	86	40	46	80.0 ± 2.0	90.0 ± 0.7	94.0 ± 3.0	65	80.0 ± 0.7
OKT9	N.D.	5	N.D.	9	2.5 ± 0.8	3.5	3.5	3.5	2.5 ± 0.8	5.1 ± 0.7	5.5 ± 2.7	2	2.5 ± 0.9
OKT10	N.D.	N.D.	N.D.	86	78.0 ± 4.0	75	95	68	83.0 ± 0.8	94.5 ± 0.7	90.0 ± 7.0	N.D.	90.0 ± 0.8
$\beta2$-m	8	21	11	N.D.	86.5 ± 6.5	97	86	85	80.5 ± 0.8	95.0 ± 1.5	94.0 ± 4.0	61	95.0 ± 1.0
OKIa1	1	1	1	1	1.8 ± 0.2	1.5	1.0	3.8	4.0 ± 0.5	3.0 ± 0.4	6.5 ± 1.1	1.3	4.0 ± 0.3
Leu-7	<0.1	<0.1	<0.1	<0.1	<0.1	<0.1	<0.1	<0.1	<0.1	<0.1	<0.1	<0.1	<0.1

[a]Percentage of positive cells as determined by flow cytometry analysis (mean ± standard duration).

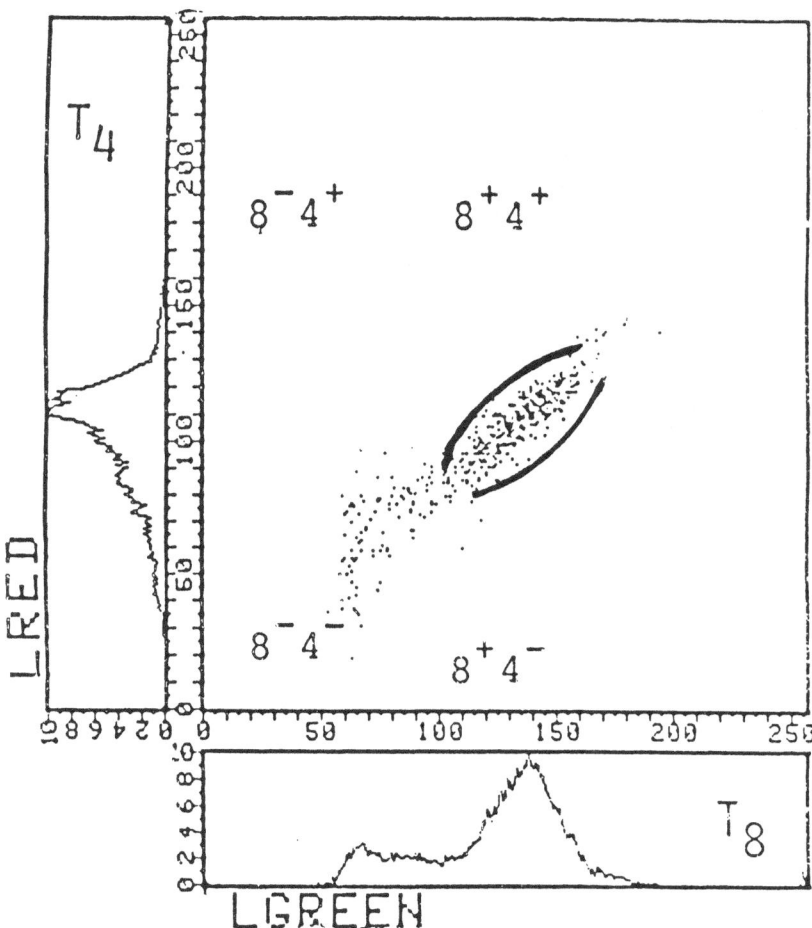

Figure 1. Flow cytometric analysis of fetal thymocytes following double immunofluorescence labeling.

with those obtained by Abo et al. [1]. They have also demonstrated that the NK activity of fetal bone marrow against K562 target cells was very weak and only detectable when the few HNK-1-positive cells were separated from the other bone marrow cells. Toivanen et al. [16] and Uksila et al. [20] have demonstrated a low but detectable NK functional activity in most livers from 9 to 23 week-old fetuses; it was increased by in vitro incubation with interferon.

Effect of α-IFN on surface markers

Following incubation of fetal mononuclear cells with α-IFN, no increased mortality and no alteration of the cell size were observed. When cells were labeled with anti-β2-m antibodies, an increase in fluorescence intensity of α-IFN-treated cells was consistently found in the three fetal organs

Table 4. Surface markers expressed by fetal spleen mononuclear cells.

MoAb	Gestational age (weeks PF)						
	14	15	16	17	20	21	25
OKT11	22[a]	42	35	46	35	47	47
OKT3	55	45	50	56	44	48	54
OKT4	23	26	32	31	23	37	28
OKT8	24	N.D.	24	21	31	34	20
OKT6	N.D.	N.D.	10	16	19	15	12
OKT9	N.D.	N.D.	16	N.D.	N.D.	21	32
OKT10	41	42	57	78	61	60	66
β2-m	N.D.	84	83	89	62	91	89
OKIa1	46	39	39	46	21	36	41
Leu-7	< 0.1	< 0.1	< 0.1	N.D.	N.D.	< 0.1	< 0.1

[a]Percentage of positive cells as determined by flow cytometry analysis.

analyzed (Table 5, 6, and 7). The expression of class I HLA molecules at the cell surface was simultaneously enhanced and this augmentation enabled us to perform HLA typing on α-IFN-treated thymocytes or spleen cells from 14 and 15 week-old fetuses [12]. The selective effect of α-IFN on histocompatibility antigens and on certain differentiation antigens was supported by the finding of an enhanced expression of T10 (Table 5) contrasting with the unmodified expression of the specific T-cell markers (T3, T4, T6, T8 and T11) at all fetal ages tested, in the fetal thymus (data not shown).

The capacity of α-IFN to increase the expression of H2 antigens in murine adult lymphocytes [9], β2-m and class I HLA antigens in human PBL [5] and HLA antigens in 18–21 week-old thymocytes [6] has already been described. Our studies have established that such a phenomenon could also exist in cells of younger fetuses, at a period when HLA density is much lower and HLA specificities are difficult to detect with conventional methods. This enhancement of HLA expression proved to be of value for readily typing fetal cadavers prior to transplantation.

Responsiveness to phytomitogens

Proliferative responses to ConA, PHA and PWM in relation with fetal age were investigated.

Fetal liver cells demonstrated a high degree of spontaneous proliferation and only a very slight response to ConA in 10-week old fetuses. In experiments involving cell separation on a discontinuous albumin density gradient, however, low density cells from 13–14 week-old fetuses exhibited a more substantial response to ConA, PHA and, to a lesser extent, PWM (data not shown).

Mitogen responsiveness of fetal thymocytes could be divided into three stages. Within the first 11 weeks of gestation, no significant thymocyte

Table 5. In vitro effect of α-IFN on the β2-m expression and the OKT10 expression on fetal thymocytes.

Gestational age (weeks PF)	β2-m-positive thymocytes				OKT10-positive thymocytes			
	Percentage of positive cells[a]		Median fluorescence intensity[a]		Percentage of positive cells[a]		Median fluorescence intensity[a]	
	0	α-IFN	0	α-IFN	0	α-IFN	0	α-IFN
7	8	20	15	42	N.D.	N.D.	N.D.	N.D.
14	86	85	22	46	79	90	69	101
15	97	96	38	61	75	95	43	89
16	86	88	25	52	95	94	56	103
17	85	90	40	96	68	100	63	128
20	93	90	64	102	94	100	67	98
21	94	98	52	105	84	98	39	71
23	61	72	40	96	N.D.	N.D.	N.D.	N.D.

[a]Determined by flow cytometry analysis.

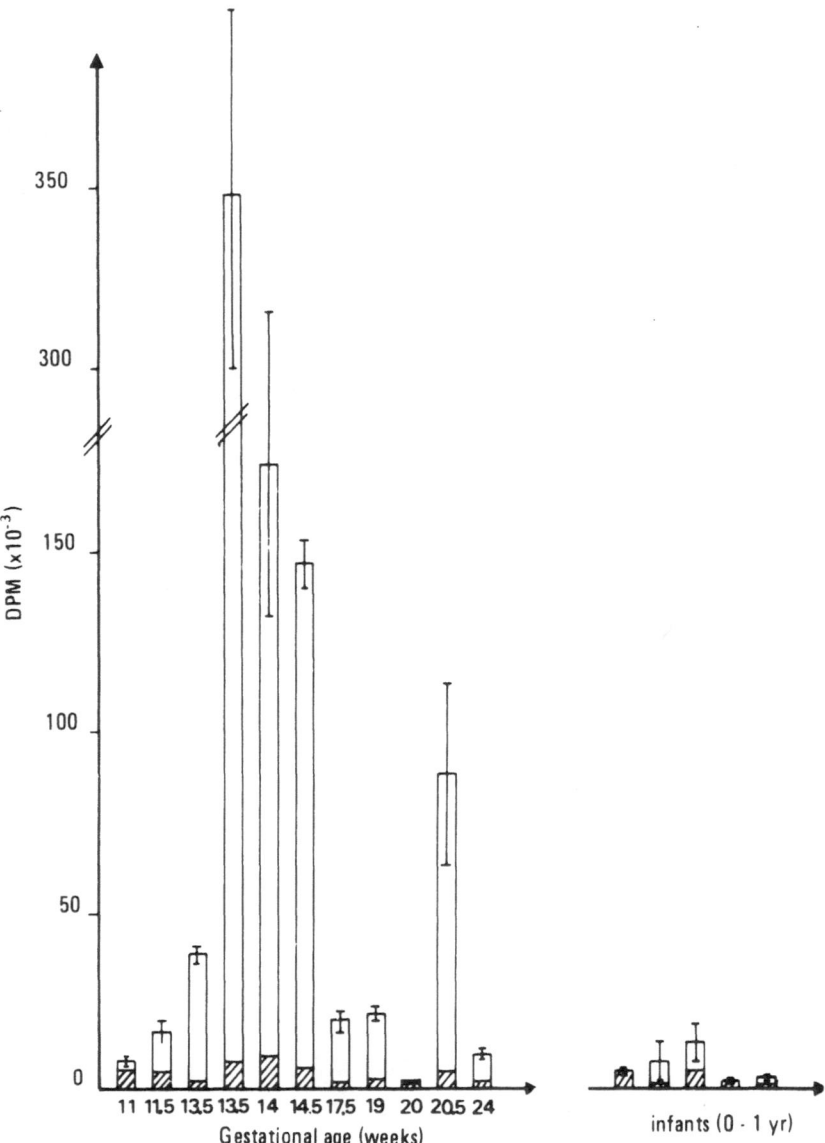

Figure 2. Proliferative response of fetal thymocytes to ConA. Analysis at different time post-fecundation (gestational age).

proliferative response to mitogen was observed. This period reflected thymus colonization with lymphoid stem cells or prothymocytes from the fetal liver (7–11 weeks). At 13–14 weeks of gestation, thymocytes became highly responsive to ConA, to PHA and to PWM (Figures 1, 2 and 3). These proliferative capacities persisted, but decreased in magnitude at 15–16 weeks of gestation. During the last period (from 16 weeks onwards),

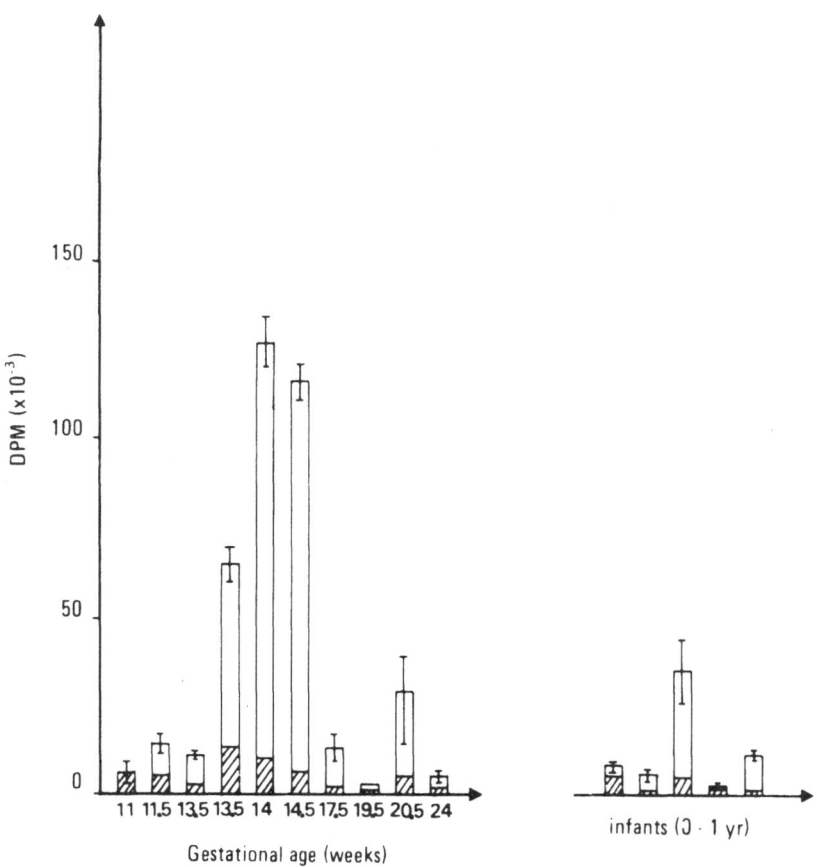

Figure 3. Proliferative response of fetal thymocytes to PHA. Analysis at different time post-fecundation (gestational age).

fetal thymocytes did not express a more significant responsiveness to mitogen stimulation than thymocytes from children did.

These results confirm the capacity of fetal thymocytes to respond to phytomitogens [14]. They further support the scheme of differentiation

Table 6. In vitro effect of α-IFN on the β2-m expression fetal liver cells.

Gestation age (weeks PF)	Percentage of β2-m positive cells[a]		Median fluorescence intensity[a]	
	0	α-IFN	0	α-IFN
7	4	12	13	31
12	17	29	20	37
13	14	19	20	82
14	10	21	11	80
15	19	26	11	41
16	26	35	39	73
21	46	50	54	120

[a]Determined by flow cytometry analysis.

68

Table 7. In vitro effect of α-IFN on the β2-m expression on fetal spleen cells.

Gestational age (weeks PF)	Percentage of β2-m-positive cells[a]		Median fluorescence intensity[a]	
	0	α-IFN	0	α-IFN
15	84	89	33	51
16	83	85	70	125
17	89	87	90	210
20	62	72	84	165
21	91	96	134	223

[a]Determined by flow cytometry analysis.

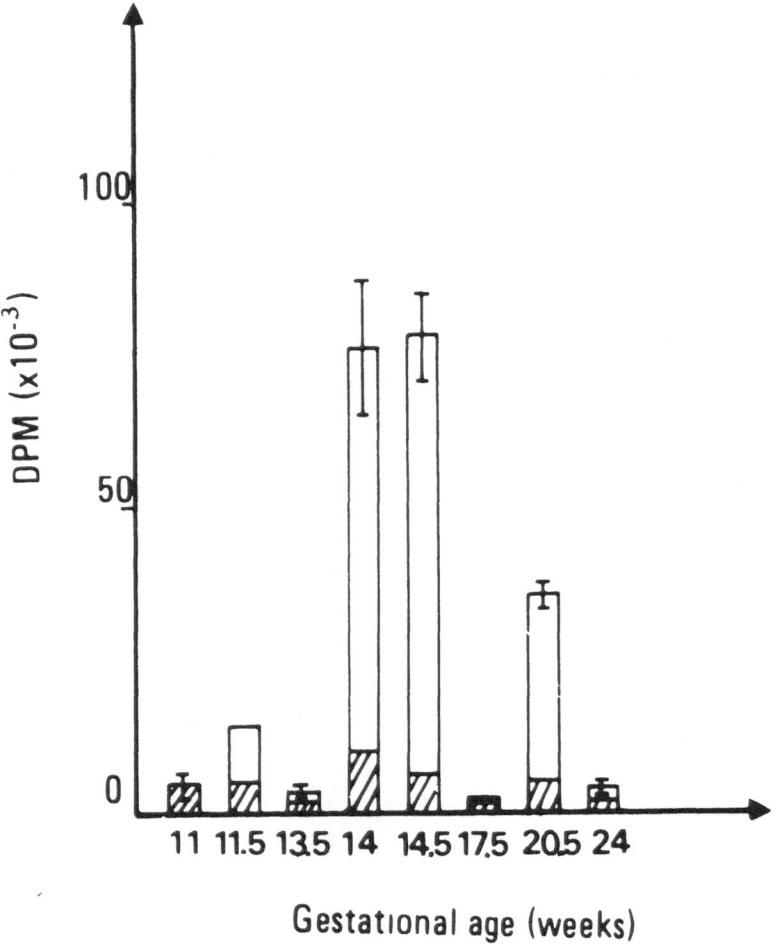

Figure 4. Proliferative response of fetal thymocytes to PWM. Analysis at different time post-fecundation (gestational age).

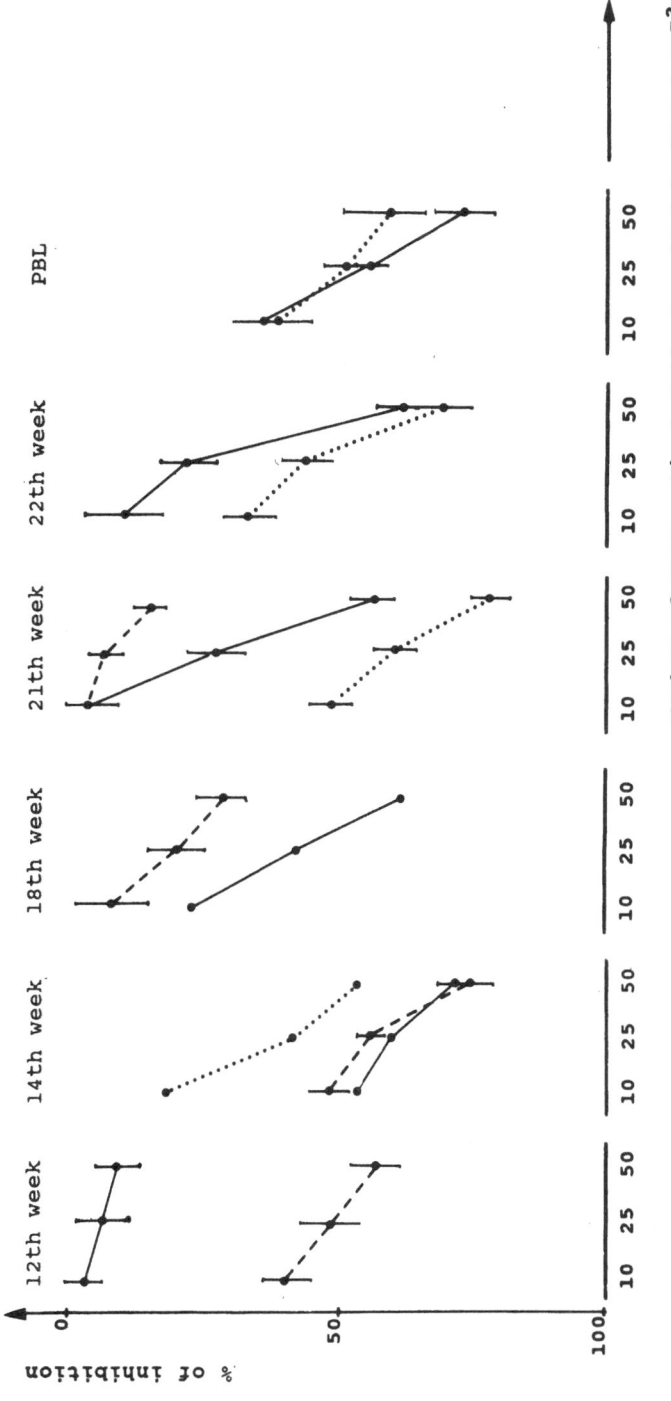

Figure 5. Suppressor activity of fetal splenocytes (——— layers 2 + 3 of BSA gradient, i.e. low density cells, · · · layer 4 of BSA gradient, i.e. high density cells), fetal thymocytes (– – –) and adult PBL (——— layers 2 + 3 of BSA gradient, i.e. low density cells, · · · · layer 4 of BSA gradient, i.e. high density cells). When several samples from the same age were investigated, the mean and the standard deviation of the percentage of inhibition were calculated.

involving the sequential appearance of mitogen responsiveness after the acquisition of certain surface markers [17]. These data also suggest some differences at distinct stages of development. Between weeks 13 and 16, a transient homing of relatively mature T-cells takes place in the thymus together with local production of IL-1, IL-2 and possibly other factors enhancing proliferative responses. After 16 weeks gestation, a large proportion of relatively mature T lymphocytes leave the thymus and complete maturation is then achieved in peripheral lymphoid organs.

The mitogen responsiveness of spleen cells was observed a few weeks after the appearance of a proliferative response of thymocytes. We could not determine distinct sequential stages at the spleen level (data not shown).

Suppressor activity

Experiments were carried out to investigate a possible suppressor activity displayed by fetal cells. The assay involved polyclonal activation of suppressor lymphocytes from the thymus or the spleen by ConA, with subsequent inhibition of proliferative response in mixed lymphocyte culture (MLC) by the ConA-activated lymphoblasts isolated on a discontinuous albumin density gradient.

From 14 weeks onwards, splenocytes exhibited some suppressor activity although sometimes at a lesser degree than did PBL in the same assay (Figure 5). Inhibition of the allogeneic response by ConA-activated thymocytes was consistently found in 14 week-old thymuses. After the 15th week, the suppressor activity appeared to be somewhat reduced in the thymus, as was the proliferative response to ConA. The part played in this assay by the degree of expression of IL-2 receptor is currently under investigation in fetal thymocytes of different ages. A suppressor activity

Table 8. Percentage of intracytoplasmic (IgM + IgG + IgA)-positive cells following incubation of the unseparated lymphoid cells from fetal liver, thymus and spleen, in the presence or in the absence of PWM.

Gestational age (weeks PF)	Fetal liver		Fetal thymus		Fetal spleen	
	0	PWM	0	PWM	0	PWM
12	0	0	0	0	0.1	0.9
13	0	0	0	0	0.1	1.0
14	0	0	0	0	0.2	1.3
16	0	0	0	0	0	2.5
17	0	0.1	0	0	0.6	4.0
18	0	0	0	0	0.3	2.2
20	0	0.1	0	0	0.3	4.0
21	0	0	0	0	0.5	3.6
23	0	0	0	0	0.5	4.4

Results in control adult PBL(n = 8) were the following:
without PWM: 0.20 ± 0.01;
with PWM: 7.0 ± 1.2

Table 9. Percentage of intracytoplasmic (IgM + IgG + IgA)-positive cells following in vitro incubation of separated and co-cultured T- and B-cells in the presence or in the absence of PWM.

| Separated cell populations | | Gestational age (weeks PF) of fetal organ | | | |
| T-cells + B-cells | | 12–14 (n = 5) | | 15–23 (n = 8) | |
		0	PWM	0	PWM
f.T[a]	—	0	0	0	0
f.S[b]	—	0.2	0.1	0	0.1
—	f.S	0.1	0.2 ± 0.1	0.1	0.3 ± 0.1
f.T	f.S	0.2	2.5 ± 0.1	0.1	3.0 ± 0.7
f.S	f.S	0.2	1.5 ± 0.5	0	3.8 ± 0.4
a.PBL[c]	f.S	0	3.7 ± 0.4	0.1	4.3 ± 0.9
f.T	a.PBL	0	3.6 ± 0.4	0.2	1.2 ± 0.4
f.S	a.PBL	0	1.9 ± 1.0	0.4	4.5 ± 0.2

[a] fetal thymcytes;
[b] fetal splenocytes;
[c] adult PBL.
Results in control adult PBL (n = 8) were the following:
— B-cells + PWM: 0.2 ± 0.06;
— T-cells + PWM: 0.0;
— T-cells + B-cells: 0.4 ± 0.1;
— T-cells + B-cells + PWM: 5.6 ± 1.4.

has also been demonstrated in the fetal liver, as early as 10 weeks, by Rabinowich et al. [10].

Helper activity

PWM is known to induce in vitro differentiation of B-cells into plasmacytoid cells with intracytoplasmic immunoglobulins, through activation of helper T-cells [8].

When unseparated lymphoid cells from the various fetal organs were incubated with PWM, this B-cell differentiation was demonstrated to occur in the spleen cell population but not in thymocytes or liver cells (Table 8). Fetal spleen, but neither thymus nor liver, contains both helper T-cells and responsive B-cells.

To check for possible helper T-cells in the fetal thymus, we co-cultured fetal thymocytes and B-cells from either adult PBL or fetal spleen in the presence of PWM. A moderate helper activity was observed, demonstrating some helper T-cells in the fetal thymus. The degree of helper activity was larger in fetal thymus than in fetal spleen at 12–14 weeks but it was larger in fetal spleen in 15–23 weeks. However, the values obtained did not quite reach those observed when T-cells and B-cells had been prepared from adult PBL (Table 9). When B-cells from the fetal spleen were cocultured with fetal helper T-cells from the spleen in the presence of PWM, an intracytoplasmic synthesis of IgM only was seen; when adult T-cells were used, fetal B-cells could synthetize not only IgM, but also IgG (Table

Table 10. Percentage of intracytoplasmic IgM-positive cells and intracytoplasmic IgG-positive cells following incubation of fetal spleen cells in the presence of PWM.

	Gestational age (weeks PF)			
	12–14 (n = 5)		15–23 (n = 8)	
	PWM IgM$^+$ cells	IgG$^+$ cells	PWM IgM$^+$ cells	IgG$^+$ cells
Unseparated fetal spleen suspension	1.0 ± 0.9	0.1 ± 0.1	3.5 ± 1.2	1.0 ± 0.8
Separated cells T-cells + B-cells				
f.S f.S	1.5 ± 0.5	0.1 ± 0.1	3.0 ± 1.0	0.6 ± 0.4
a.PBL f.S	2.2 ± 1.0	1.8 ± 0.3	2.9 ± 0.6	1.2 ± 0.0

Same legend as in Table 9.
Results in control adult PBL (n = 8) were the following:
  unseparated cells + PWM: 4.4 ± 0.3 IgM$^+$;
              3.0 ± 1.1 IgG$^+$;
  T-cells + B-cells + PWM: 4.3 ± 1.3 IgM$^+$;
              2.4 ± 1.9 IgG$^+$.

10). These data suggest that fetal T-cells have some, but not all, functional helper capacities of adult T lymphocytes.

Conclusion

The immunological analysis of lymphoid cells from human fetuses has shown that most T-cell markers and T-cell functions are acquired between the end of the first trimester and the end of the second one. This is also the time of very intensive proliferation, resulting in a dramatically increased number of cells of the T lineage. Much before the 24th week, this large population of T-lymphocytes, although not yet fully mature in every respect, does possess the capacity to induce a very strong and rapid GvHD following transplantation into an immunodeficient and allogeneic host.

Transplants of fetal livers less than 13–14 weeks of age do not carry a major risk of severe acute GvHD, since T-cells are very scarce at this period in the liver. A transitory homing of relatively mature T-cells has been noticed in the thymus after the 13th week and, for this reason, it seems to be advisable to irradiate fetal thymus cells of more than 12 weeks when they are to be transplanted into immunodeficient patients, in order to prevent acute GvHD.

Whether or not fetal T-cells can exert as potent reactivities against common antigens as they are known to exist against histocompatibility determinants still has to be more fully investigated. Preliminary results suggest that the gene rearrangement leading to the expression of the T-cell receptor takes place in the thymus at a relatively early stage and that fetal T-cells are equipped to recognize antigen and initiate a response to it before the end of the second trimester.

References

1. Abo T, Miller CA, Gartland GL, Balch CM (1983) Differentiation stages of human natural killer cells in lymphoid tissues from fetal to adult life. J. Exp. Med. 157:273.
2. Asma GEM, Langlois Van Den Bergh R, Vossen JM (1983) Use of monoclonal antibodies in a study of the development of T lymphocytes in the human fetus. Clin. Exp. Immunol. 53:429.
3. Boyüm A (1968) Isolation of mononuclear cells and granulocytes from human blood. Scand. J. Clin. Lab. Invest. 21 (suppl. 97), 9:109.
4. Carr MC, Stites DP, Fudenberg HH (1973) Dissociation of response to phytohemagglutinin and adult allogeneic lymphocytes in human foetal tissues. Nature New Biol. 241:279.
5. Fellous M, Kamoun M, Gresser I, Bono R (1979) Enhanced expression of HLA antigens and B2-microglobulin on interferon-treated human lymphoid cells. Eur. J. Immunol. 9:446.
6. Hockland M, Ritsz J, Hockland P (1983) Interferon-induced changes in expression of antigens defined by monoclonal antibodies on malignant and non-malignant mononuclear hematopoetic cells. J of Interferon Research, 3:199.
7. Janossy G, Tidman N, Papageorgiou ES, Kung PC, Goldstein G (1981) Distribution of T lymphocyte subsets in the human bone marrow and thymus: An analysis with monoclonal antibody. J. Immunol. 126:1608.
8. Keightley RG, Cooper MD, Lawton AR (1976) The T cell dependence of B-cell differentiation induced by Pokeweed Mitogen. J. Immunol. 117:1538.
9. Lindahl P, Leary P, Gresser I (1974) Enhancement of the expression of histocompatibility antigens of mouse lymphoid cells by interferon in vitro. Eur. J. Immunol. 4:779.
10. Rabinowich H, Beharay C, Ben-Aderet N, Klajman A (1983) Cellular and humoral suppressor activity induced by Concanavalin A-stimulated human fetal liver cells. Transplantation 35:452.
11. Reinherz EL, Kung PC, Goldstein G, Levy RH, Schlossman SF (1980) Discrete stages of human intrathymic differentiation: Analysis of normal thymocytes and leukemic lymphoblasts of T-cell lineage. Proc. Natl. Acad. Sci. USA 77:1588.
12. Royo C, Touraine JL, Bétuel H (1985) HLA-typing of fetal cells using interferon treatment in vitro. In: Gale RP, Touraine JL, Lucarelli G (eds) Progress in Clinical and Biological Research, Fetal Liver Transplantation. New York: Alan R. Liss, Inc., 193:149.
13. Siegal FP, Siegal M, Good RA (1976) Suppression of B-cell differentiation by leukocytes from hypogammaglobulinemic patients. J. of Clin. Invest. 58:109.
14. Stites DP, Carr MC, Fudenberg HH (1974) Ontogeny of cellular immunity in the human fetus: Development of responses to phytohemagglutinin and to allogeneic cells. Cellular Immunol 11:257.
15. Streeter GL (1920) Foot length of the foetus. Contributions to Embryology 11:143.
16. Toivanen P, Uksila J, Leino A, Lassila O, Hirvonen T, Ruuskanen (1981) Development of mitogen responding T-cells and natural killer cells in the human fetus. Immunol. Rev. 57:89.
17. Touraine JL, Hadden JW, Good RA (1977) Sequential stages of human T lymphocyte differentiation. Proc. Natl. Acad. Sci. USA 74:3414.
18. Touraine JL, Touraine F, El Mohandes A, de Bouteiller O, Salle B (1980) Suppressor T lymphocytes active on mixed lymphocyte reaction in man: Stage of differentiation of suppressor T lymphocytes. In: Transplantation and Clinical Immunology. Amsterdam: Excerpta Medica 12:121.
19. Touraine JL, Roncarolo MG, Royo C, Touraine F (1987) Fetal tissue transplantation, bone marrow transplantation and prospective gene therapy in severe immunodeficiencies and enzyme deficiencies: Thymus, this issue.
20. Uksila J, Lassila O, Hirvonen T, Toivanen P (1983) Development of NK cell function in the human fetus. J. Immunol. 130:153.

Thymus 10:75–87 (1987)
© Martinus Nijhoff Publishers, Dordrecht

Fetal tissue transplantation, bone marrow transplantation and prospective gene therapy in severe immunodeficiencies and enzyme deficiencies

J.-L. TOURAINE,[1] M.G. RONCAROLO, C. ROYO and F. TOURAINE

Transplantation and Immunobiology Unit, Pavillon P, Hôpital Edouard Herriot, F-69437 Lyon Cedex 08, France

(Accepted 19th May 1987)

Key words: Human, transplantation, fetal liver, fetal thymus, bone marrow, stem cells, gene transfer, immunodeficiencies, inborn errors of metabolism

Summary. The successful development of fetal tissue transplantation has resulted in therapeutical solutions for patients with a variety of diseases. Fetal liver transplants as well as bone marrow transplants, can completely cure patients with severe combined immunodeficiency disease. These transplants can also be applied to treat other types of immunodeficiency, hemopathies, and inborn errors of metabolism, in association with immunosuppressive therapy. Despite complete HLA incompatibility between transplanted stem cells and host cells, functional activities of donor-derived T-lymphocytes are not restricted. In severe forms of Di George syndrome, immunological reconstitution can be obtained by fetal thymus transplantation. It is expected that, in the near future, pure stem cell transplants and gene transplants will develop and will provide remarkable solutions for the therapy of a large number of diseases.

Introduction

Severe combined immunodeficiency diseases (SCID) are relatively heterogeneous conditions with a spontaneously fatal outcome due to infections, usually before one year of age. Patients with SCID can be completely cured by bone marrow transplantation (BMT), especially from an HLA genotypically-identical donor [2, 5, 8].

When no compatible donor is available, the patients can receive either an haplo-identical BMT or a fetal liver transplant (FLT). In the first alternative, the bone marrow must be treated in vitro to eliminate every T-lymphocyte able to induce or enhance a graft-versus-host disease (GvHD). In the second alternative, the fetal liver is best used in combination with the thymus from the same donor, and the optimal age for the fetal donor is 8–12 weeks following fecundation. In both cases, the

---

[1] Author for correspondence.

immunological reconstitution develops more slowly than following an HLA-identical BMT. Complete isolation in sterile 'bubbles' is therefore mandatory.

Since 1974, we have performed 101 fetal liver and/or thymus transplants in 38 patients: eleven SCID infants have been treated by fetal liver and thymus, twenty-one patients with inborn errors of metabolism received fetal livers, five infants with Di George syndrome and one patient with Bare Lymphocyte syndrome had a thymus transplant.

Bone marrow transplantation in SCID

In our transplant center, seven patients with SCID have been treated by BMT (Table 1). In each case, the donor was an HLA-identical sibling and $1.5-2.5 \times 10^8$ nucleated bone marrow cells per kg of body weight were used. Three patients received one transplant and four received two transplants a few months apart. Graft 'takes' was obtained in all seven patients. Two patients died at 1 and 4 months respectively, due to previous conditions, and five patients are alive, healthy, and cured of their disease. All five patients have full immunological reconstitution, stable for 1–12 years.

One of the two deaths was due to previous BCG infection and the severity of such generalized BCG infections in patients with SCID has already been reported [20]. No improvement of the patient's condition was observed despite the attempt at immunological reconstitution associated with anti-TB antibiotics. The other death was the result of malabsorption and hypoglycemia in a patient who had many episodes of gastroenteritis before BMT [18].

The five patients with full immunological reconstitution are four boys and one girl.

The previously described incidence of complications in the host using female donors [1] was not encountered in this series. One moderate and

Table 1. HLA-identical bone marrow transplantation in 7 patients with SCID (Lyon, 1974–1986).

Patient	Treatment	Take	GvHD	Reconstitution	Outcome
T (male)[a]	BMT (sister)[b]	+++	+	Full	Complete recovery
C (female)	BMT (sister)	+++	(+)	Full	Complete recovery
M (male)	BMT (sister)	+++	−	Full	Complete recovery
H (female)	BMT (brother)	++	−	Initial	Death (previous BCG infection)
D (male)[b]	BMT (brother)	+++	−	Initial	Death (malabsorption and hypoglycemia)
S (male)	BMT (brother)	+++	−	Full	Complete recovery
C (male)	BMT (brother)	+++	−	Full	Complete recovery

[a]Patient with ADA deficiency;
[b]Patient with Bare Lymphocyte syndrome;
[c]BMT = 1 or 2 bone marrow transplants per patient.

one very mild GvHD developed in these infants and they recovered spontaneously. The first infant had a GvHD following a blood transfusion performed before the diagnosis of SCID was suspected. A BMT from an HLA-identical sister was performed soon afterwards, resulting in the disappearance of GvHD and of previous infections. A skin rash and a moderate liver involvement were observed after one week, but they disappeared rapidly and spontaneously. A second BMT from the same donor was not followed by any skin manifestation. In this patient, it is believed that the transplanted cells have permitted elimination of the transfused lymphocytes which were responsible for the GvHD. BMT may therefore contribute to the cure of GvHD.

Ideally, the diagnosis of SCID should be made at birth and BMT performed immediately. It is then a very simple procedure which can almost be conducted in the outpatient clinic. BMT should not, however, be denied to severely infected patients, provided that antibiotics and other measures to control infection are, at least partially, effective before BMT. Except for one patient with a family history of SCID, who was treated soon after birth, all patients subjected to BMT in our institution had previously had severe infections, including pneumocystis and candida infections. These infections were cured by antibiotics and immunological reconstitution, without sequellae.

Following BMT, differentiation markers and functions of T-lymphocytes developed progressively over the first three to six months. OKT8 + cells increased rapidly in peripheral blood, while OKT4 + cells remained relatively limited in number for the initial three months. Immunoglobulin levels rose progressively, especially after the second month. Frequently, immunoglobulins (particularly IgG) of restricted heterogeneity were detected during a transient phase, followed by immunoglobulins of normal heterogeneity. Four to six months were usually necessary before a completely normal spectrum of immunoglobulin classes and subclasses was obtained, at which time antibody production was also normal.

The origin of various cells has been determined using chromosomal markers, especially in BMT across a sex barrier. In every case, T-lymphocytes derived from donor cells. In SCID patients without B-cells, B-lymphocytes also developed from donor cells, although a little more slowly than T-lymphocytes. In SCID patients with B-cells, most of peripheral blood B-lymphocytes remained of host origin, contrasting with the donor origin of T-cells. It is worth of note that class I and class II HLA antigens were identical in host and donor, therefore identical on B cells and T cells. Monocytes and macrophages have not been studied in every case; they seem to derive in large part from host stem cells. Similarly PMN leukocytes and erythrocytes remained of host type.

Some SCIDs are the result of primary enzyme deficiency. The more documented and, for the time being, the more frequently detectable enzyme defect leading to SCID is adenosine deaminase (ADA) deficiency. It is known that ADA deficiency hinders development of lymphocytes, especially T-lymphocytes [11], but whether or not other cells or tissues are altered by ADA deficiency can only be answered by prolonged follow-up of patients with ADA deficiency in whom lymphocytes only are replaced by normal cells. In such a male patient treated twelve years ago by BMT from his HLA-identical and ADA-heterozygous sister, we have observed a specific reconstitution of the T-lymphocyte population by cells of donor origin, with XX chromosomes. B-lymphocytes, PMN leukocytes, erythrocytes and apparently all other cells remained of host type. Only T-lymphocytes had increased ADA activity, at an heterozygous level (as all the sister's cells). Besides full reconstitution of cellular and humoral immunities, all physiological functions have been normal. In particular, bones and cartilages, which initially showed minimal lesions [11], developed normally. The reconstitution of a T-cell compartment with ADA-positive cells was sufficient for a complete cure of the consequences of this enzyme deficiency.

Without doubt, BMT from a genotypically HLA-identical sibling is, at present, the best and most satisfactory treatment of SCID. It results in rapid reconstitution and complete recovery, and no additional treatment is necessary. When γ-globulins and antibiotics are given before the transplant and during the initial follow-up, they can be discontinued after a few months. In most SCIDs, no conditioning is necessary prior to transplantation. In a few cases (e.g., some ADA-deficient patients) the 'take' may be difficult or insufficient, and a conditioning regimen prior to transplantation can then be useful. GvHD, when it occurs, is mild or moderate, with a favorable outcome, in these SCID patients treated by HLA-identical BMT.

In over 60% of patients, however, no perfectly compatible donor can be found in the family. The choice is then between an incompletely compatible BMT and an FLT. An haplo-identical BMT can be carried out provided that all GvHD-inducing T-lymphocytes are removed from the transplanted bone marrow. Several methods have been developed to achieve T-cell depletion of bone marrow: rosetting with sheep erythrocytes, fractionation with soybean-agglutinin, treatment with one or several anti-T-cell monoclonal antibodies. Experience with these methods has resulted in progressively improved results. A number of problems, however, are still awaiting solutions: decreased incidence of 'take' following T-cell depletion of the graft, split chimerism, incomplete immunological reconstitution, occurrence of EBV-induced B-cell lymphomas, occasional persistence of some donor T-cells, etc. [4, 9, 12, 14, 15]. When T-cell depletion may be insufficient, treatment of the patient with ciclosporine may be helpful. When graft failure is feared, heavy immunosuppression prior to BMT or repeated administration of anti-LFA-1 monoclonal

Table 2. Fetal liver and thymus transplantation in 11 patients with SCID (Lyon 1976–1986).

Patient	Treatment	Take	GvHD	Reconstitution	Outcome
S (male)	FLTT[b]	+ + +	–	Full	Complete recovery
B (male)[a]	FLTT	?	–	No	Death (previous BCG infection)
C (female)	FLTT	+ + +	–	Full	Complete recovery
F (female)	FLTT	+ +	+ +	Partial	Death (meningitis)
M (male)	FLTT	+	+ + +	Initial	Death (GvHD and septicemia)
M (male)	FLTT	+ + +	–	Full	Complete recovery
M (male)	FLTT	+	+ +	Initial	Death (infection with Salmonella and catheter complications)
T (female)	FLTT	+ +	+ (chronic)	Almost complete	Recovery from immunodeficiency
B (male)	FLTT	+ +	–	Almost complete	Recovery from immunodeficiency
T (male)	FLTT	?	–	No	Early death (hemorrhages and renal failure)
B (male)	FLTT	+	–	Still partial	Healthy, still in hospital

[a]Patient with ADA deficiency;
[b]FLTT = 1 to 8 fetal liver and thymus transplants per patient.

antibody can be used: these maneuvres increase the incidence of graft take, but unfortunately they also increase the frequency of infectious complications. In a recent European survey [4], it has been shown that 57.1% of patients treated with T-cell-depleted haplo-identical BMT were alive after 2 years; among these alive patients a little less than 50% had a complete T-cell and B-cell reconstitution.

Fetal liver and thymus transplantation in SCID

When no HLA-identical donor was available for BMT, we always resorted to fetal liver and thymus transplantation (FLTT) for the treatment of SCID patients. We have treated 11 SCID patients with this mode of therapy (Table 2). Stem cells from the fetal liver can proliferate and differentiate after transplantation in the host, resulting in lymphocyte repopulation and immunological reconstitution. Because of their immaturity, stem cells confronted by allogeneic antigens acquire immunological tolerance to these antigens. When the stem cell suspension is devoid of lymphocytes already engaged in T-cell differentiation, no GvHD can occur initially. Following differentiation of some stem cells into T-lymphocytes, no or only minimal GvHD occurs.

It is suggested that the immune reconstitution provided by FLT is enhanced by simultaneous transplantation of thymus from the same donor [3, 13] which provides a syngeneic environment for T-lymphocyte differentiation of transplanted stem cells. Such an FLTT does not appear

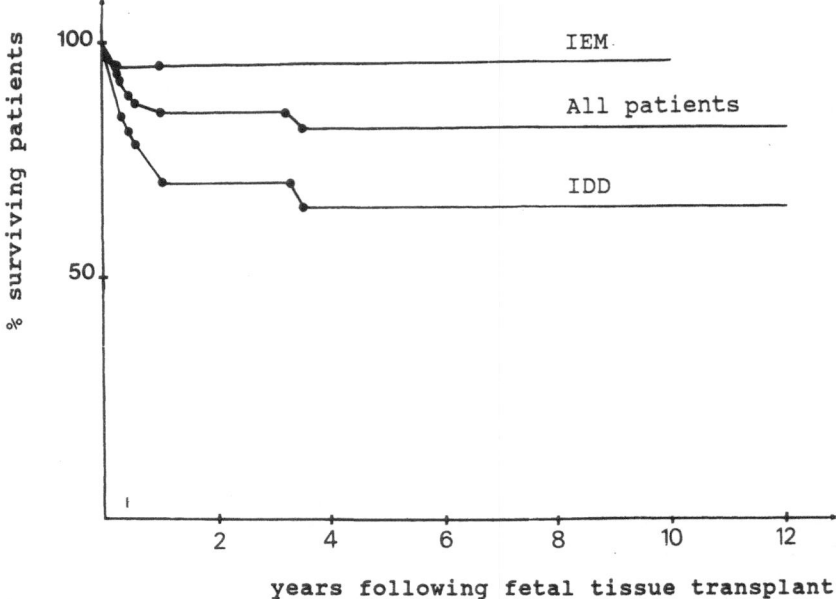

Figure 1. Patient survival over the years after fetal tissue transplantation. The median curve represents all patients, including both the patients with inborn errors of metabolism (IEM) and those with immunodeficiency diseases (IDD).

to result in an increased risk of GvHD [3], at least when the thymus is at an early stage of fetal development.

For the above-mentioned reasons, we have used FLTT from 8 to 13 week-old (post-fecundation age) fetuses, in all 11 patients. Thymuses which contained numerous thymocytes, i.e. 13 week-old thymuses, were irradiated with 4000 rads prior to transplantation. The transplant consisted of the intraperitoneal injection or intravenous infusion of a suspension of fetal liver and thymus cells. A part of the cell suspension was also injected intramuscularly in the first three patients. Only fresh fetal tissues were used and the viability of all cell suspensions was found in every case to exceed 70%, as evaluated by the trypan blue method. The mean number of cells transplanted from an individual fetus was 8.2×10^8 nucleated cells, i.e. 1.3×10^8 per kg of body weight.

No attempt at HLA matching of the donor and the recipient was made.

The patients received 1 to 8 sequential FLTTs. Our initial approach was to repeat FLTT five months after the first FLTT only if results were felt to be insufficient. At present, we carry out a systematic series of eight FLTTs a few days apart on each patient, a method which does not seem to have drawbacks, but which increases the probability of graft 'take' from at least one of the transplants.

All patients were isolated in sterile 'bubble' and decontaminated as much as possible prior to FLTT; isolation was prolonged until virtually full reconstitution was obtained, no matter how long this process took. One boy was left for 1.5 years in the isolator and one girl for 3.5 years. Adaptation of these young children to their limited environment has been remarkable and no significant psychological problem has been encountered either during isolation or after their removal from the 'bubble'.

Five patients died due to previous BCG infection, to GvHD associated with septicemia, to resistant Salmonella infection, to neurologic sequellae of meningitis, and to hemorrhages associated with renal failure, respectively. Six patients are alive and very healthy (Figure 1). Five of them have an immunological reconstitution. They lead completely normal lives, at home, and are off therapy for 3 to 10 years after the transplant. The last patient, recently treated, is still in hospital, but no longer in isolation since his immunological reconstitution has significantly progressed over the last few weeks (Table 2).

Graft take could easily be documented by identification of cells with an HLA phenotype different from that of the host. HLA-typing also allowed determination of which of the sequential transplants had taken: the first FLTT in two patients, one of the further FLTTs in the others. Moderate GvHD occurred in four patients, transplanted with fetal tissues less than 13 weeks old. Two GvHDs improved under prednisone treatment but the previously existent infection led to death. Another GvHD was virtually cured by prednisone, but neurological sequellae following meningitis led to death more than three years after FLTT. The fourth GvHD, of chronic type and mild intensity, was controlled by the treatment (Table 2).

Immunological reconstitution has developed progressively, but it was much slower than that after HLA-identical BMT. In the patients attaining full reconstitution, it developed over approximately two years [21], stressing the need for decontamination and perfectly sterile isolation. If not isolated, patients with SCID treated by FLTT would not survive long enough for the development of immune defenses against micro-organisms. After two years, in the above-mentioned patients, the numbers of T-lymphocyte, their subsets, the proliferative responses to various stimuli, and the T-cell cytotoxic responses were virtually normal. Immunoglobulin levels, allohemagglutinins and antibody production following vaccination approached normal after three years only. IgG were first of restricted heterogeneity, then normal.

The first child had the following HLA phenotype: HLA A3 A33 B14 B47 DR4 DR5. The fetal donor from whom reconstituting cells derived (second donor) was HLA A1 A2 B18 B27 DR1 DR7. No HLA A, B or DR specifity was therefore shared by donor and recipient. By separation of T- and B-lymphocyte populations, followed by HLA-typing, it was demonstrated that all T-lymphocytes were of donor origin, while B-lymphocytes were of host origin. The monocyte population included two varieties of cells: a few monocytes derived from donor cells, most of them

82

Table 3. Favorable factors in FLT.

Patient	
— Early diagnosis, isolation and treatment — Lack of infection	— Prolonged isolation in sterile environment
Transplant	
— Fresh fetal tissue — Fetal donor 8–12 weeks of age — Repeated transplants (2–8) — No. of nucleated cells > 10^8/kg of body weight of recipient	— i.p. or i.v. route? — Male donor? — Syngeneic thymus associated to liver?
Role of compatibility?	

from host cells. Despite complete HLA mismatch at the A,B and DR loci, T-lymphocytes of donor origin could, in particular, recognize tetanus toxoid antigen presented by host monocytes and help host B-lymphocytes for antitetanus toxoid antibody synthesis in vitro [16]. They also exerted effector functions on various other host cells. Defense against virus infections in vivo was normal and T-cell cytotoxic functions were present in vitro toward a large variety of target cells. It was noteworthy that, in this patient, T-lymphocytes had differentiated from stem cells in the context of both donor and host antigens, due to the presence of the two thymuses.

Comparable findings were obtained in the study of the other patients reconstituted by FLTT, demonstrating the efficacy of this form of therapy.

From a review of these cases, as well as from other reports, some factors could be defined as favorable for the outcome of the FLT (Table 3). The respect of such conditions lead to results virtually as good with FLTT as with HLA-identical BMT, in patients with SCID. Whether or not the addition of fetal thymus transplant to FLT is definitely beneficial in man is still uncertain, since we never used FLT alone in these infants.

The 'Allo + X' hypothesis

In contrast with predictions [23], we observed that, following the slow reconstitution induced by FLTT, no important restriction of T-cell function was imposed by either donor or host MHC. T-cell cytotoxic responses toward target cells with a variety of MHC-determinants were present. In addition, T-cells did co-operate with HLA-mismatched monocytes and B-cells, in an antibody production system.

Although we could not determine whether donor stem cells differentiated into host or donor thymus, these results suggested that the restriction of T-cell response by the MHC may not be absolute in human transplantation. Several explanations for this lack of significant restriction in long-term human chimeras can be postulated [17]: (a) partial in vivo restriction when more absolute restriction appears to exist in vitro by lack of very discriminative assay; (b) absolute restriction in short experiments as in the mouse, but a partial one in long-term T-cell reconstitution; (c) restriction partially imposed by the thymus MHC, partially by the lymphoid-cell MHC; (d) absolute restriction in inbred animals, but a partial one in outbred individuals, in which many cross-reactions between MHC determinants have been demonstrated; (e) possibility to circumvent the restriction, e.g. by progressive development of allo + X recognition ('allo + X' hypothesis).

The apparent discrepancy between experimental data and results in patients following allogeneic FLTT does not appear to result from a species difference nor from a major difference between inbred and outbred individuals. Even in classic, inbred mice, evidence is now accumulating to suggest that restriction is not a systematic, absolute phenomenon, but rather reflects a relative 'preference' of T-cells for syngeneic cells in several types of interactions. When recognition of self + X is not proposed to T-cells, alternative mechanisms of recognition (possibly of the 'allo + X' type) may develop.

The 'allo + X' hypothesis [19, 21] has been based on the following facts: (a) in most models where MHC restriction has been unequivocally demonstrated, the control experiments with allogeneic target cells show a low, but present, response; (b) in our chimeric patients, T-cells become progressively capable of all types of interaction with allogeneic host cells: (c) in circumstances where MHC restriction is not observed, MHC products are still necessary, suggesting that the presence of these molecules at the surface of target cells is important even when they are of a different specificity [10].

In the thymus there may be development of T-cell subsets, each of which has a primary recognition structure for a given type of histocompatibility antigens. In normal circumstances, only those T-cells with recognition for self-histocompatibility antigens are solicited (because the allo-antigens are not encountered); these cells are induced to proliferate and to develop the full repertoire of antigen recognition in association with self-recognition. In chimeric patients, a given set of other histocompatibility antigens is also continuously presented to T-cells. Those T-cells with recognition for the given alloantigens are then solicited, they expand by proliferation and develop the gene rearrangement leading to the expression of the T-cell receptor. Antigen recognition is then associated with alloantigen recognition. Whether, in these chimeric patients, 'self + X' and 'allo + X' recognitions are supported by the same or by distinct T-cells is a question that we analyzed by developing T-cell clones from these patients. The results showed that T-cells recognizing antigen in the context of allo-specificities are found in high frequency, in these patients, and they have no recognition ability for self + X.

The crucial role of class I and class II HLA antigen presentation to T-lymphocyte precursors in the thymus is suggested by the severe immune incompetence of patients with the Bare Lymphocyte syndrome [18]. The lack of expression of either class I or class II HLA antigens in this condition results in the inability of T-lymphocytes to develop the repertoire of antigen recognition.

Fetal thymus transplantation in Di George syndrome

Fetal thymus transplantation (FLTT) has also been used as a treatment for patients with severe forms of the Di George syndrome. We have performed FTT in 5 such patients. One of them died of severe cardiopathy. Two patients had a full and rapid immunological reconstitution, as well as clinical recovery, stable after 1 and 12 years. Two recently treated patients still have a partial — but progressing — immunological reconstitution (follow-ups < 6 months).

Fourteen other patients with more partial forms of Di George syndrome and less severe immunodeficiency were treated with thymic factor administration or other forms of therapy.

Fetal liver transplantation in inborn errors of metabolism

A variety of inborn errors of metabolism (IEM), without associated immunodeficiency, have been treated by FLT, in conjunction with a prolonged immunosuppressive therapy at moderate doses (comparable to those given in non-severe auto-immune diseases). No adverse effect was seen. Patient survival is shown in Figure 1. The diseases treated were the following: Gaucher, 4; Fabry, 4; Fucosidosis, 2; Hurler, 2; Metachromic leucodystrophy, 2; Hunter, 1; Glycogenosis, 1; San Filippo B, 1; Morquio B, 1; Niemann-Pick A, 1; Niemann-Pick B, 1; and Niemann-Pick C, 1.

Two of the patients died of their initial disease and one is currently in hospital. The other patients are in relatively good condition and display objective criteria of partial improvement [21]. The serum levels of the defective enzymes were not dramatically increased, but the various substrates measured were decreased and tissue deposits were stabilized. By contrast with immunodeficiencies treated by FLT or FTT, these patients have only a partial and usually transient benefit of this mode of therapy. In many of them, FLT had to be repeated after some months or after a few years. Donors selected for FLT in IEM were relatively older than those chosen for FLTT in SCID. The respective part played by the stem cells and by the hepatocytes in the improvement seen after FLT is currently under investigation. The viability of the transplanted fetal liver cells could be monitored using the sequential measure of serum α-fetoprotein (AFP). Following FLT, AFP levels rose sharply, then decreased progressively while cells matured in 1–2 months.

Table 4. Some characteristics of BMT, FLT and SC transplants (SCT).

	Allog.BMT	FLT	SCT
Donor-recipient compatibility	required	not required	not required
GvHD	+++ (reduced by T-cell depletion)	(±)	(±)
Transmission of harmful virus	+++	(±)	(±)
Search for donor	sometimes tedious	sometimes tedious	easier
Ethical problems associated with cell procurement	++	++	(±)

Isolated stem cell transplantation

It is our belief that, in the future, both BMT and FLT, as they are presently performed, will be replaced by purified stem cell transplants [22], together with appropriate growth and differentiation factors. The availability of stem cell cultures, especially developed from fetal livers, would be advantageous in many respects: immediate accessibility for all patients, no tedious search for donor, no need for matching, little risk of GvHD or of harmful virus transmission (Table 4). We are now able to maintain fetal liver stem cells in culture for more than two months, but several problems remain to be solved: identification of culture conditions and of growth factors that can lead to significant multiplication of stem cells without in vitro differentiation; determination of the optimal number of stem cells to transplant and of the immunsuppressive conditioning to use when the patient has some residual immunity; development of methods increasing the rapidity for a full reconstitution.

Gene transplantation in immunodeficiencies and inborn errors of metabolism

Insertion of functioning gene into deficient cells is becoming an alternative to allogeneic cell transplantation in some IEM. The ADA deficiency, which results in SCID, may be an appropriate candidate for the development of this new therapy. Correction of the gene defect in hematopoietic stem cells, and therefore in lymphocytes, will cure the disease following restitution of those stem cells to the patient. The human ADA gene has been cloned and can be inserted in vitro into human and sub-human primate cells, using a retrovirus-mediated gene transfer system [6, 7]. These cells can be infused back in an animal, by autologous transplantation [6]. Because ADA-corrected lymphocytes will probably have a selective advantage in their further development, their proportion may increase with time. In most experiments carried out till now, however, gene expression could be maintained to a certain degree in the in vitro cultures, at least for some time, but tended to decrease substantially following the in vivo cell transfer. There are thus some problems to be solved, but it is reasonable to assume that gene transplantation will soon be ready for application to some of the well-defined gene defects in man.

Conclusion

BMT has been successfully developed as a therapy of immunodeficiency diseases since 1968. It also represents now a very efficient treatment of leukemia, aplastic anemia and other hemopathies. A little later, FLT proved its capacity to cure SCID, without any need for histocompatibility. Its application to other diseases is feasible. In the future, these forms of treatment may be replaced by transplantation of pure stem cells, together with appropriate growth and differentiation factors. Transplantation of allogeneic stem cells, in particular produced in culture from fetal liver, and gene transfer combined with autologous marrow transplantation, will probably establish their value in the field of immunodeficiencies then, as BMT and FLT did, will expand into many other areas of medicine.

Acknowledgment

We are grateful to G. Souillet, B. Bétend, N. Philippe, R. Francois, H. Bétuel, A. Paris, J. Banchereau, H. Spits and J. de Vries for help in care of the patients and in some of the in vitro studies. France-Transplant and Biogref organizations contributed to fetal tissue procurement, in accordance with the rules of the Ethical Committee.

References

1. Bortin MM, Gale RP, Rimm AA (1981) Allogeneic bone marrow transplantation for 114 patients with severe aplastic anemia. Jama 245:1132.
2. Bortin MM, Rimm AA (1977) Severe combined immunodeficiency disease: Characterization of the disease and results of transplantation. Jama 238:591.
3. Bortin MM, Salzstein EC (1969) Graft-versus-host inhibition: Fetal liver and thymus cells to minimize secondary disease. Science 164:316.
4. Fischer A, Griscelli C, Friedrich W, Kubanek B, Levinsky R, Morgan G, Vossen J, Wagemaker G, Landais P (1986) Bone marrow transplantation for immunodeficiencies and osteopetrosis: European Survey, 1968–1985. Lancet 2:1080.
5. Gatti RA, Allen HD, Meuwissen HJ, Hong R, Good RA (1968) Immunological reconstitution of sex-linked lymphopenic immunological deficiency. Lancet 2:1366.
6. Gillio A, Bordignon C, Kantoff P, Eglitis M, McLachlin J, Kernan N, Karson E, Zwiebel J, Gilboa E, Anderson WF, O'Reilly R (1986) Retrovirus mediated transfer of the human ADA gene into primate hematopoietic cells and subsequent in vivo expression following autologous bone marrow transplantation. Presented at the International Congress of Immunology, Toronto.
7. Kahn DB, Kantoff P, Mitsuya H, Eglitis M, Gilboa E, Anderson WF, Blaise RM (1986) Reconstitution of lymphoid cells from adenosine deaminase (ADA)-deficient SCID

patients by an ADA-retroviral vector gene transfer system. Presented at the International Congress of Immunology, Toronto.

8. Koning J de, Van Bekkum DW, Dicke A, Dooren LJ, Van Rood JJ, Radl J (1969) Transplantation of bone marrow cells and fetal thymus in an infant with lymphopenic immunological deficiency. Lancet 1:1223.

9. Levinsky RJ, Davies EJ, Linch D, Goldstone AH, Beverly PCL (1982) Soybean lectin fractionation of bone marrow to prevent graft-versus-host disease (GvHD) in mismatched transplants. Exp. Hematol. 10 (Suppl 10):96.

10. Lipinski M, Fridman WH, Tursz T, Vincent C, Pions D, FellousM (1979) Absence of allogeneic restriction in human T-cell mediated cytotoxicity to Epstein-Barr virus infected target cells: Demonstration of an HLA-linked control at the effector level. J. Exp. Med. 150:1310.

11. Meuwissen HJ, Pickering RJ, Pollara B, Porter IH (1975) Combined Immunodeficiency Disease and Adenosine Deaminase Deficiency: A molecular Defect. Academic Press: New York.

12. O'Reilly RJ, Kapoor N, Kirkpatrick D, Flomenberg N, Pollack MS, Dupont B, Good RA, Reisner Y (1985) Transplantation of hematopoietic cells for lethal congenital immunodeficiencies: In Primary Immunodeficiency Diseases, Birth Defects. The National Foundation March of Dimes 19:129.

13. Pahwa R, Pahwa S, Good RA, Incefy GS, O'Reilly RJ (1979) Rationale for combined use of fetal liver and thymus for immunological reconstitution in patients with variants of severe combined immunodeficiency. Proc. Natl. Adac. Sci. USA 74:3002.

14. Prentice HG, Blacklock HA, Janossy G, Bradstock KF, Skeggs D, Goldstein G, Von Hoffbrand V (1982) Use of anti-T-cell monoclonal antibody OKT3 to prevent acute graft-versus-host disease in allogeneic bone marrow transplantation for acute leukemia. Exp. Hematol. 10 (Suppl. 10):99.

15. Reisner Y, Kapoor N, Pollack S, Dupont B, Chagant RSK, Good RA, O'Reilly RJ (1981) Transplantation for acute leukemia with HLA-A and B non identical parental bone marrow cells fractionated with soybean agglutinin and sheep red-blood cells. Lancet 2:327.

16. Roncarolo MG, Touraine JL, Blanchereau J (1986) Cooperation between major histocompatibility complex mismatched mononuclear cells from a human chimera in the production of antigen-specific antibody. J. Clin. Invest. 77:673.

17. Touraine JL (1980) Cooperation between thymus and transplanted precursor cells during reconstitution of immunodeficiencies with bone marrow or fetal liver cells. In: Thierfelder S, Rodt H, Kold HJ (eds) Immunobiology of Bone Marrow Transplantation p. 141. Springer: Berlin.

18. Touraine JL (1981) The Bare Lymphocyte Syndrome: Report on the Registry. Lancet 1:319.

19. Touraine JL, Bétuel H (1981) Immunodeficiency diseases and expression of HLA antigens. Human Immunology 2:147.

20. Touraine JL, Philippe N, Bétuel H, Souillet G, Bétend B, Souteyrand P, Schmitt D (1981) GvHR and infectious complications in SCID patients treated by bone marrow or fetal liver. In: Touraine JL, Gluckman E, Griscelli C (eds) Bone Marrow Transplantation in Europe, Vol. 2 p. 209. Excerpta Medica: Amsterdam.

21. Touraine JL (1983) Bone marrow and fetal liver transplantation in immunodeficiencies and inborn errors of metabolism: Lack of significant restriction of T-cell function in long-term chimeras despite HLA-mismatch. Immunol. Rev. 71:103.

22. Touraine JL, Royo C, Murray K, Roncarolo MG, de Bouteiller O (1987) Will bone marrow transplantation be eventually replaced by unmatched stem cell transplantation? Bone Marrow Transplantation (in press).

23. Zinkernagel RM (1978) The thymus: Its influence on recognition of 'self-major-histocompatibility antigens' by T-cells and consequences for reconstitution of immunodeficiency. Springer Semin Immunopathol 1:405.

Thymus 10:89–94 (1987)
© Martinus Nijhoff Publishers, Dordrecht

Fetal liver transplantation in aplastic anemia and leukemia

ROBERT PETER GALE

Department of Medicine, Division of Hematology and Oncology, UCLA School of
Medicine, Los Angeles, CA 90024, USA

Summary. This study reviews results of fetal liver transplantation in hematologic disorders
including aplastic anemia, leukemia and thalassemia. One hundred and twenty two patients
received transplants for aplastic anemia; engraftment was reported in 4 patients; graft-
versus-host disease (GvHD) did not occur. Complete and partial responses were reported in
one-half of patients, the majority of whom had no evidence of engraftment. Thirty-nine
patients received transplants for leukemia. Transient engraftment was reported in 40% and
two developed GvHD; survival extended to more than 2 years. The higher rate of engraftment in patients with leukemia suggests a role of pretransplant immune suppression. The risk
of GvHD appears to be low despite complete HLA-mismatching. These data suggest a
possible role for fetal liver transplantation in man. Future studies should probably be based
on preclinical data obtained in large animal models.

Fetal liver cells are a source of hematopoietic stem cells with decreased
immune reactivity [reviewed in 1, 2]. These observations have led to
limited trials of fetal liver transplantation in patients with immune and
genetic diseases and hematologic disorders including aplastic anemia and
leukemia. In this chapter I briefly review the current status of fetal liver
transplantation in hematologic diseases.

A review of fetal liver transplantation in man was performed using data
bases from CANCERLIT, MEDLARS, and MEDLINE of the National
Library of Medicine. Data were analyzed with regard to total patients,
fetal age, number of cells transplanted, pre-transplant conditioning, engraftment, evidence of engraftment, graft-versus-host disease (GvHD),
disease response and survival. Some reports were inadequate for critical
analysis for several reasons. Individual patients were frequently not identified and many patients received more than one fetal liver transplant;
approximatey one-third of transplants consisted of multiple fetal livers.
One major obstacle to critical analysis of these data was the lack of
convincing evidence of fetal liver cell engraftment in most cases. For
example, immune reconstitution does not necessarily indicate engraftment. Other studies reported engraftment based on the demonstration of
new HLA antigens on recipient lymphocytes, of donor type red blood cell
antigens or of hemoglobin F expression. These data are problematic
because recipients are frequently extensively transfused and because fetal

hemoglobin synthesis can occur in the setting of bone marrow recovery following chemotherapy or irradiation.

Results of fetal liver transplantation in aplastic anemia are reviewed in Table 1 [3–10]. One hundred and twenty-two patients received transplants between 1960–1986; approximately one-half had severe aplastic anemia. Age of fetal donors was 6–32 weeks; most were below 20 weeks. Total dose of nucleated fetal liver cells of hematopoietic origin was $0.004–13 \times 10^8$. Six patients received cyclophosphamide pre-transplant; 115 received no pre-transplant immune suppression; one individual was exposed to 8.2 Gy total body irradiation in a reactor accident.

Four of 122 patients (3%) were reported to have grafts; in all instances this was transient. Engraftment was documented by cytogenetic analyses in 3 cases. In one patient no convincing data were presented. None of the 4 patients developed GvHD. Complete or partial responses occurred in 66 patients (54%); survival ranged from less than 1 to over 10 years.

Results of fetal liver transplantation in acute leukemia are reviewed in Table 2 [6, 10–12]. Thirty-nine patients received transplants for acute leukemia between 1978–1986. Twenty-seven had acute myelogenous leukemia (AML) and 12, acute lymphoblastic leukemia (ALL). In 23 patients, pre-transplant immune suppression was cyclophosphamide (60–120 mg/kg) and total body irradiation (5–10 Gy). Sixteen patients were receiving induction chemotherapy with daunorubicin and cytarabine for AML followed by fetal liver infusions.

Sixteen of 36 patients (41%) were reported to have transient grafts. Long-term engraftment was reported in 2 cases [6, 10]. Transient engraftment was documented by chromosome analyses in 12, RBC isoenzymes or antigens in 5, HLA antigens in 2 and HbF synthesis in 3. Two patients developed mild GvHD. Survival ranged from less than 1 to over 2 years. Since in this setting antileukemic effect is generally attributed to chemotherapy and/or irradiation, it is not possible to determine if outcome or response is related to the transplantation of fetal liver cells.

Several important conclusions emerge from these data. First, it is possible to achieve at least transient hematopoietic engraftment following transplantation of fetal liver cells. This has been rather convincingly demonstrated by cytogenetic analyses in 12 cases of acute leukemia. The incidence of successful engraftment was higher in patients with leukemia than those with aplastic anemia (41% vs. 4%). In the 23 leukemia patients who received intensive pre-transplant immune suppression, the incidence of engraftment was 54%. These data are consistent with data in rodents, dogs and man which indicate that fetal liver cells are immunogenic and likely to be rejected following transplantation to immune competent recipients. Patients with aplastic anemia generally have an intact immune system and would be expected to be at high-risk of rejecting fetal liver cells. Leukemia patients, both because of their disease and because of the use of

Table 1. Fetal liver transplantation in aplastic anemia.

Author	No.	Fetal age (w)	No. cell ($\times 10^8$)	Conditioning	Graft	Evidence	GvHD	Response	Survival (m)	Ref
Scott	14	NI	20–200	–	1	NI	No	2	4–146+	3
Keleman	1	6	0.4	–	No	–	–	1	52+	4
O'Reilly	1	10–14	15	+	No	–	–	1	52+	5
Izzi	5	10–25	0.8–13	+	No	–	–	1	<1->36+	6
Kochupillai	40	8–32	0.004–11.1	+(1)	3	Chr(3)[6]	No	22	<1–106	7, 8
Lou	60[1]	–	–	–	–	–	–	38[2]	–	9
Wu	1[3]	18	120	+	NE[5]	–	No	1	–	10
TOTAL	122	6–32	0.004–13	7	4(3%)	–	–	66(54%)	<1–146+	

[1] "Chronic" aplastic anemia, 56; acute, 4.
[2] Responses in 36/56 chronic, 2 of 4 acute.
[3] Radiation accident exposure 5.2 Gy.
[4] NI, not indicated
[5] NE, not evaluable
[6] Chr — Chromosomes

Table 2. Fetal liver transplantation in acute leukemia.

Author	No.	Fetal age (w)	No. cell (× 10⁸)	Conditioning	Graft	Evidence	GvHD	Survival (m)	Ref
Izzi	13	12–22	0.3–7	+	4	Chr(3), RBC(1), HbF(3)	No	<1–27 +	6
Kochupillai	16	10–24	0.07–39	+	2	Chr(1), RBC(1)	No	<1–32	11
Wu, Meng	10	21–24	5.6–81	+	8	Chr(7), RBC(1)	2	5–28 +	10, 12
TOTAL	39	10–24	0.3–81	39	14(36%)		2	<1–32	

high-dose, pre-transplant chemotherapy and irradiation are less likely to reject their grafts.

Graft rejection or failure of engraftment remains the major obstacle to fetal liver transplantation in man. There are several reasons why fetal liver cells are likely to be rejected. First, relatively few hematopoietic stem cells are transplanted. Second, fetal liver transplants contain few, if any, T-lymphocytes. T-cells appear to be important in obtaining sustained engraftment. Several mechanisms may be operative, including a direct interaction with hematopoietic stem cells, a graft-anti-host immune response, and possibly by serving a source of excess donor antigen to direct host anti-donor response. Bone marrow transplants depleted of T-cells are at increased risk of graft-rejection. In a recent analysis of approximately 400 HLA-matched, T-cell depleted bone marrow transplants the incidence of graft rejection was 15% compared to 1% in recipients of non-T-cell depleted grafts. The risk of rejection is even higher in non-matched cases: 30% in 100 recipients of HLA-partially matched, T-cell depleted bone marrow transplants. Because of these considerations it is not surprising that failure of engraftment and rejection are common following fetal liver transplantation. In dogs and preliminary clinical trials more intensive pre- and post-transplant immune suppression, with higher doses of radiation, and post-transplant use of methotrexate and cyclosporine [13–16] results in decreased risk of graft rejection. Most recipients of fetal liver transplants received doses of drugs or radiation which would not be expected to result in sustained engraftment over HLA-identical bone marrow cells.

GvHD has not been a major problem following fetal liver transplantation in man. It is not possible to know if this relates to the immune incompetence of the fetal liver cells or to the high incidence of graft failure. This issue will need to be addressed when a higher rate of successful, sustained engraftment is achieved. A second consideration is the possibility of an increased risk of leukemia relapse following transplants of fetal liver cells. This appears to occur in recipients of T-cell depleted bone marrow transplants [17].

In summary, there has been progress in applying fetal liver transplantation to hematologic diseases in humans. The major problem is achieving sustained engraftment. Recent data in dogs suggests that this may be achievable with more intensive pre- and post-transplant immune suppression. When results in these animal models are optimized, it may be reasonable to apply these approaches to humans.

Acknowledgment

Supported in part by grant CA 23175 NCI, NIH, USPHA, DHHS. Data in this manuscript were updated to include presentations at a symposium

94

on New Directions in Fetal Liver Transplantation. New Delhi, 1–5 February 1986. Drs. Wu and Kochupillai kindly provided their data which are detailed in the accompanying manuscripts.

References

 1. Fetal Liver Transplantation: Current Concepts and Future Directions: Lucarelli G, Fliedner TM, Gale RP (eds). Excerpta Medica, Amsterdam, 1980
 2. Fetal Liver Transplantation: Gale RP, Touraine J-L, Lucarelli G (eds). AR Liss, New York, 1985
 3. Scot RB, Matthias JQ, Constandoulakis M, Kay HEM, Lucas PF, Whiteside JD: Hypoplastic anemia treated by transfusion of fetal hematopoietic cells. Brit Med J 2:1385, 1961
 4. Kelemen E: Recovery from chronic idiopathic bone marrow aplasia of a young mother after intravenous injection of unprocessed cells from the liver (and yolk sac) of her 22 mm CR-length embryo. Scand J Haemat 10:305, 1973
 5. O'Reilly RJ, Pahwa R, Kagan W, Kapoor N, Sorell M, Meyers P, Good RA: Reconstitution of hematopoietic function in post-hepatic aplasia following high-dose cyclophosphamide and allogenic fetal liver transplantation. In: Lucarelli G, Fliedner TM, Gale RP (eds) Fetal Liver Transplantation: Current Concepts and Future Directions. Excerpta Medica, Amsterdam, 1980. pp.
 6. Izzi T, Polchi P, Galimberti M, et al.: Fetal liver transplantation in aplastic anemia and acute leukemia. In: Gale RP, Touraine J-L, Lucarelli G (eds) Fetal Liver Transplantation. AR Liss, New York, 1985, pp. 237
 7. Kansal V, Sood SK, Batra AK, et al.: Fetal liver transplantation in aplastic anemia. Acta Haemat 62:128, 1979
 8. Kochupillai V, Sharma S, Francis S, et al.: Bone marrow reconstitution following human fetal liver infusion (FLI) in sixteen severe aplastic anemia patients. In: Gale RP, Touraine J-L, Lucarelli G (eds) Fetal Liver Transplantation. AR Liss, New York, 1985, pp. 237
 9. Lou FD, Liu HC, Wang YZ: Short-term and multiole fetal liver transplantation (FTL) for treatment of aplastic anemia: Report of 15 cases. Chinese J Intern Med 24:65, 1985
10. Wu C-T, Ye G-Y: Advances in experimental studies and clinical application of fetal liver cells. Thymus, this issue
11. Kochupillai V, Sharma S, Francis S, Mehra NK, et al.: Fetal Liver Infusion: An adjuvant in the therapy of acute myeloid leukemia (AML). In: Gale RP, Touraine J-L, Lucarelli G (eds) Fetal Liver Transplantation. AR Liss, New York, 1985, pp. 267
12. Meng P-L, Fei R-G, Gu D-W, Yie W-Z: Allogenic fetal liver transplantation in acute leukemia. In: Gale RP, Touraine J-L, Lucarelli G (eds) Fetal Liver Transplantation. AR Liss, New York, 1985, pp. 281
13. Stitzel KA, Champlin RE, Gale RP: Fetal liver transplantation in dogs: A possible alternative source of hematopoietic cells for transplantation. In: Gale RP (ed) Recent Advances in Bone Marrow Transplantation. AR Liss, New York, 1983, pp. 831
14. Champlin RE, Cain G, Stitzel K, Gale RP: Fetal liver transplantation in dogs: Results with DLA-compatible and incompatible grafts. In: Gale RP, Touraine J-L, Lucarelli G (eds) Fetal Liver Transplantation. AR Liss, New York, 1985, pp. 195
15. Prummer O, Werner C, Raghavachar A, Nothdurft W, Calvo W, Steinbach K-H, Fliedner TM: Fetal liver transplantation in the dog. Transplantation 40:498, 1985
16. Prummer O, Calvo W, Fliedner TM: Variation of treatment conditions alters the outcome of fetal liver transplantation in dogs. Submitted
17. Mitsuyasu RT, Champlin RE, Gale RP, Ho WG, et al.: Treatment of donor bone marrow with monoclonal anti-T cell antibody and complement for the prevention of graft-versus-host disease: A prospective randomized double blind trial. Submitted

Thymus 10:95–102 (1987)
© Martinus Nijhoff Publishers, Dordrecht

Fetal liver infusion in aplastic anaemia

V. KOCHUPILLAI,[1] S. SHARMA,[1] S. FRANCIS,[1] A. NANU,[2] S. MATHEW,[3]
P. BHATIA,[1] H. DUA,[1] L. KUMAR,[1] S. AGGARWAL,[1] S. SINGH,[1] S. KUMAR,[4]
A. KARAK[5] and M. BHARGAVA[5]

[1] Medical Oncology Department, Institute Rotary Cancer Hospital, [2] Blood Bank,
[3] Cytogenetic Laboratory, [4] Obstetrics and Gynaecology Department, [5] Pathology
Department; All India Institute of Medical Sciences, New Delhi, IND-110 029, India

Key words: fetal liver infusion, severe aplastic anaemia, haemopoietic reconstitution

Summary. Forty patients with severe aplastic anaemia received an intravenous infusion of
0.004 to 11.1 × 10^8 (median: 8 × 10^8) hematopoietic cells prepared from the fetal livers of
8–32 week old abortuses. Five patients, who died within 15 days of fetal liver infusion, are
excluded from analysis. Twenty-two of the 35 evaluable patients (62%) responded favour-
ably. Six of the 7 patients with good response were alive after 9 to 44 months (median:
m = 20); one died 106 months after fetal liver infusion due to renal lithiasis. Four of the 7
with moderate response were alive after 9 to 31 months; 3 died within 16 months. Of 8
patients with minimal response, one was lost to follow-up and the others died in 3.4 to 10
months (m = 6). Median survival of responders was 15.7 months. Bone marrow cellularity
became normal in 12 patients following fetal liver infusion. In seven patients, there was a
relapse; 6 regained a normal bone marrow cellularity after a second or third fetal liver
infusion. These data strongly suggest a role of fetal liver infusion in inducing bone marrow
recovery. Of 13 non-responders, 4 were lost to follow-up and 9 died within 20 days–4.3
months (m = 1.6). Fetal liver infusion appears to be an effective therapy in patients with
severe aplastic anaemia.

Introduction

Conservative therapy including blood component transfusion, androgens
and/or corticosteroids may benefit 50–75% of individuals with mild or
moderate aplastic anaemia [7, 15, 23, 26]. Severe aplastic anaemia, however, usually does not respond to these measures [9, 15]. Two major
approaches used to treat patients with this condition, are bone marrow
transplantation and antithymocyte globulin (ATG) administration. In
bone marrow transplantation, the recipient is immuno-suppressed, then
transplanted with matched allogeneic stem cells. ATG therapy, for reasons
as yet unclear, promotes recovery of the patient's own bone marrow. Both
approaches have limitations. Allogeneic bone marrow transplantation
requires an expensive and sophisticated infra-structure and an HLA-
matched donor. Complications such as graft-vs-host disease (GvHD) and
interstitial pneumonia occur in a significant proportion of transplant
recipients [8]. ATG is expensive and of limited availability.

Address for offprints: Dr. Vinod Kochupillai, Associate Professor of Medical Oncology,
Institute Rotary Cancer Hospital, All India Institute of Medical Sciences, New Delhi, IND
— 110 029, India.

Fetal liver is an alternative source of haematopoietic stem cells. Infusion of fetal liver cells has recently been used in animals [4, 19] and in humans with severe aplastic anaemia, resulting in encouraging, though preliminary, results [12, 14, 16, 21, 25, 28]. In this study, we present our experience with 40 patients with aplastic anaemia who received fetal liver cell infusion. Parts of this work have been previously reported [4, 12, 13, 16, 17].

Patients and methods

From September 1976 to May 1985, 40 consecutive patients with severe aplastic anaemia received fetal liver infusion. Two of them had pure red cell aplasia and one had a normocellular bone marrow with peripheral blood pancytopenia. Thirty-five patients had severe aplastic anaemia according to previously published criteria [15] and 2 had moderate aplastic anaemia. Prior therapy included androgens in variable doses for 1–12 months (m = 3) in 27 patients; and prednisolone in 13 patients, 10 of whom also received androgens. No patient responded to these therapies. One patient received cyclophosphamide 25 mg/kg for 3 days prior to fetal liver infusion. Ten patients received no therapy prior to fetal liver infusion. With the exception of one patient, all received 1–79 blood transfusions (m = 12) prior to fetal liver infusion.

There were 36 males and 4 females. Ages ranged between 7 and 70 years (m = 23.5). Presenting symptoms included fever in 22, bleeding in 32 and both in 21 patients. The duration from diagnosis to fetal liver infusion varied from 2 days to 64 months (m = 1 month).

Etiology

Four patients had a history of ingestion of analgesics, 3 were exposed to chloramphenicol. Two patients had a history of infectious hepatitis. Two patients had pure red cell aplasia and one, dyskeratosis congenita. No etiology was identified in 28 cases.

Haematological parameters prior to fetal liver infusion

Range and median of haematological parameters at diagnosis, and one day before fetal liver infusion, in all patients except the two with pure red cell aplasia are shown in Table 1. Bone marrow biopsy revealed marked hypocellularity in 37 patients, pure red cell aplasia in 2, and normal cellularity in one.

Fetal liver infusion

Fifty-nine fetuses of 8–32 weeks (m = 16) of gestation were obtained from the Department of Obstetrics. These fetuses were available following hysterotomy in 34 cases, prostaglandin injection in 21, syntocinon drip in

Table 1. Haematological values at diagnosis and one day before fetal liver infusion.

	At diagnosis range (median)	One day before fetal liver infusion range (median)
Hb (grams/dl)	2.3–8.6 (5.1)	2.9–9.9 (5.1)
Reticulocytes (%)	0.1–4.0 (0.45)	0–3.6 (0.2)
Granulocytes (No. per μl)	0–1482 (487)	0–1716 (286)
Platelets (No. per μl)	10,000–90,000 (28,000)	10,000–120,000 (30,000)

2 and spontaneous abortion in 2. Fetal liver cell suspension was prepared, as previously described [16], and was infused intravenously within 2–240 hours. Each fetal liver infusion consisted of cells from a single fetus and each patient received cells from one fetus at a dose of 0.004–11.1 $\times$ 10^8 (m = 8 $\times$ 10^8).

Those patients with no response or with relapse after an initial response received fetal liver infusion on more than one occasion. Twenty-six patients received a single fetal liver infusion, 10 patients received 2 infusions, 3 received 3 infusions and one patient received 4 infusions. A sex difference between donor and recipient was present in 22 instances; in 32 cases, donor and recipient were of identical sex. In 5 fetuses, the sex was not recorded. To avoid possible GvHD, 28 patients received prednisolone 40 mg daily or on alternate days after fetal liver infusion. This was tapered over 1–14 months (m = 6). Twelve patients received no therapy after fetal liver infusion, except for folic acid. As there was no significant difference of the responses in these 2 groups, both are analyzed together.

Assessment of engraftment

Detailed studies of engraftment following fetal liver infusion are reported elsewhere in this volume [3]. These studies included bone marrow cultures for chromosome analyses, HLA A, B & C typing and analyses of RBC antigens and alpha-fetoprotein. Fetal hemoglobin, Hb A2 and serum iron were estimated by standard techniques [6].

Results

Response and survival

Five patients died within 15 days after receiving fetal liver infusion and are excluded from further analysis. Twenty-two of 35 evaluable cases (62%) responded. The response was slow for all haematological parameters including increase of bone marrow cellularity; the augmentation of platelets was the slowest and more often incomplete. Responses were therefore categorized as good, moderate, minimal or absent based on the degree of increase in Hb level and granulocyte count after fetal liver infusion (Table 2).

98

Table 2. Response criteria.

	Hb (grams/dl)	Granulocytes (No. per μl)
Good response	> 10	> 2000
Moderate response	8 to $\leqslant$ 10	1500 to $\leqslant$ 2000
Minimal response	6 to $\leqslant$ 8	1000 to $\leqslant$ 1500
No response	< 6	< 1000

Bone marrow cellularity generally correlated well with the response in peripheral blood counts [2]. Among 22 responders, 7 patients had a good response and all are surviving at 9–44 months (m = 20), with the exception of one patient who died 106 months after fetal liver infusion due to complications of renal stones. Seven patients had a moderate response with a median survival (MS) of 10 months; 4 are surviving to-day at 9–31 months and 3 patients died within 16 months. Eight patients had a minimal response: 1 was lost to follow-up and the others died in 3.4 to 10 months (m = 6). Thirteen patients failed to respond: 4 were lost to follow-up and 9 died in 20 days to 4.3 months (m = 1.6 month).

From the survival curve of the 22 responders (Figure 1) it can be calculated that MS among responders is 15.4 months. The probability of survival at 6 months is 75%, at one year 54%, and at 2 years it is 43%.

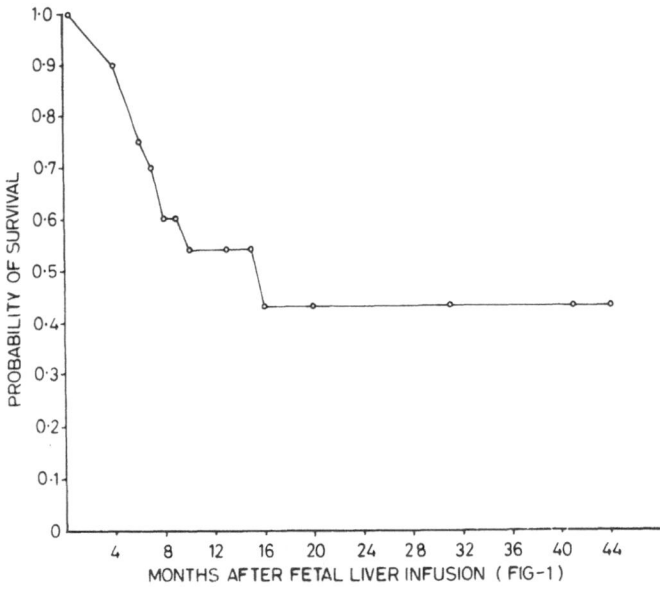

Figure 1. Actuarial survival curve for 22 responders following fetal liver infusion.

Biochemical parameters

There was a decrease in serum iron values among responders in 3–34 months (m = 4) following fetal liver infusion, indicating better utilization of iron by the bone marrow. There was a mild increase in blood sugar, serum alkaline phosphatase and SGOT in 5 days to 29 months (m = 7 months) after fetal liver infusion. Blood sugar values returned to near normal in 3–22 months (m = 15) although these did not normalize. Serum alkaline phosphatase and SGOT values remained high. There was a milder rise in the level of SGPT but no significant rise in serum bilirubin after fetal liver infusion.

Fetal haemoglobin (HbF) and Hb A2

There was a rise in fetal Hb level (1.2–9.7; m = 7.3%) in 5 of the 7 patients studied 1−19 months after fetal liver infusion. Hb A2 levels did not change after fetal liver infusion.

Assessment of prognostic factors

Factors like age, difference in donor and recipient sex, duration of symptoms at the time of fetal liver infusion, level of Hb, granulocytes, platelets and reticulocytes, number of fetal liver cells infused, fetal liver cell viability, time interval between abortion and fetal liver infusion, type of abortion, number of blood transfusions prior to fetal liver infusion and degree of dyserythropoiesis in fetal liver cells were assessed to see if these factors influenced response and survival following fetal liver infusion. None of these factors emerged as important statistically.

Evidence of engraftment

There was no significant change in HLA A, B and C, nor in red cell antigens after fetal liver infusion. No increase in the level of alpha-fetoprotein was noted. Studies of chromosomes revealed a mixture of XX and XY cells in 3 male patients. This chimerism was temporary and repeated bone marrow cultures in one patient revealed only XY metaphases. These 3 patients required a second fetal liver infusion.

Discussion

Severe aplastic anaemia is associated with high mortality rate; median survival is less than 6 months with conservative management [20]. Response rate of 60% and a median survival of 15.4 months following fetal liver infusion is a significant improvement over survival achieved with conservative management [15]. Improvement after fetal liver infusion was evidenced by an increase in peripheral blood counts and bone marrow cellularity, and decrease in blood transfusion requirement and serum iron.

The response following fetal liver infusion differs from that reported following bone marrow transplantation where haematological improvement including normal peripheral blood counts and bone marrow cellularity occurs within 3–4 weeks. After fetal liver infusion, haematological recovery is slow and not always complete. A similar response pattern has been reported following ATG therapy [30].

Cellularity became normal in 50% of patients with hypocellular bone marrow in 1–12 months (m = 6). In 7 patients, this recovery was transient; 6 of the 7 responded to a second and/or a third fetal liver infusion. Repeated responses after each fetal liver infusion suggest that improvement is related to fetal liver infusion. In the remaining 50% of patients there was partial or minimal improvement in bone marrow cellularity. Improvement is unlikely due to the addition of prednisolone in 28 patients after fetal liver infusion of whom 19 responded, since 7 of these patients had received prednisolone prior to fetal liver infusion and had not responded. It is possible that the immune suppression induced prior to fetal liver infusion might increase the response rate. One patient received cyclophosphamide 3 days before fetal liver infusion; he developed extensive pulmonary infection and haemorrhages, and he expired 22 days later. O'Reilly and coworkers, however, observed a beneficial effect of the immune suppression preceding fetal liver infusion in one case [25].

Except for 3 patients who showed temporary mixed chimerism, none of the responders had evidence of engraftment. This is supported by absence of changes in HLA or RBC antigens and alpha-fetoprotein. Of the 12 patients treated with fetal liver infusion, without pre-conditioning, by Lucarelli and coworkers [21], 2 showed engraftment evidenced by the persistent modification of red cell enzymes.

These data suggest that engraftment is not the likely mechanism of the benefit in most aplastic anaemia patients receiving fetal liver infusion. It is possible that fetal liver cells may stimulate haemopoiesis in the recipient by an as yet unknown mechanism.

Mismatched bone marrow infusion that fails to establish engraftment is known to improve aplastic anaemia in some patients [24, 30, 31]. In this connection, Nissen and coworkers [24] have postulated that transient partial chimerism, which may escape detection, could have an effect in 'rattling up' the immune system, and be responsible for the recovery of autologous bone marrow which is a slower and more incomplete process than bone marrow recovery by successful engraftment of the allogeneic bone marrow transplant. Possibility exists that fetal liver cells may contain a growth factor capable of stimulating the patients haematopoietic stem cells.

Haematopoiesis in the fetal liver is predominantly erythroid with erythroid-myeloid ratios exceeding 25:1 [5,27,29]. In contrast, myelopoiesis predominates in adult bone marrow (E:M ratio = 1:3). Patients who recover after fetal liver infusion have shown erythropoiesis as the more dominant response in the bone marrow [2,16,18]. In this connection, Alter and coworkers [1] suggested that haematopoiesis during bone marrow recovery may be associated with recapitulation of ontogeny. The fetal liver growth pattern of the bone marrow recovery as well as the rise of fetal hemoglobin, in 5 patients of the present study support this suggestion.

We noted mild increases in blood glucose, alkaline phosphatase, SGOT and SGPT following fetal liver infusion. With the exception of one patient with HBsAg positive hepatitis, no other patient had clinical symptoms. The reason for these mild biochemical abnormalities is unclear and in the absence of evidence of engraftment is unlikely to be due to overt GvHD.

The present study suggests that fetal liver infusion is an effective therapy in severe aplastic anaemia. This procedure is of particular value in countries with limited resources where bone marrow transplantation cannot be undertaken easily. Fetal liver infusion may also be of value when an HLA-matched donor is not available [10,11]. The present study indicates that more than 50% of patients who received fetal liver infusion recover from bone marrow failure. The mechanism of this recovery is unclear.

Acknowledgements

We are grateful to the Department of Science and Technology, Government of India for financing this study and to Dr Robert P. Gale, Associate Professor of Medicine, University of California in Los Angeles, USA for his useful suggestions in the preparation of this manuscript. Miss Vandana typed the manuscript.

References

1. Alter BP, Rappaport JH, Huisman THS, Schroeder WA, Nathan DG (1976) Fetal erythropoiesis following bone marrow transplantation. Blood 48:843–853
2. Bhargava M, Karak AS, Sharma S, Kochupillai V: Bone marrow recovery following fetal liver infusion (FLI) in aplastic anaemia: Morphologic studies. Thymus (this issue)
3. Bhatia P, Kochupillai V, Mathew S, Mehra NK, Nanu A, Jayasuryan N, Sharma S, Francis S.: Studies on engraftment following fetal liver infusion. Thymus (this issue)
4. Bortin MM, Rimm AA, Rose WC, Trutt RG, Saltzstein (1976) Transplantation of hematopoietic and lymphoid cells in mice. Transplantation 21:331–336
5. Cappellini MD, Potter CG, Wood WG (1984) Long term haemopoiesis in human fetal liver cell culture. Br J Haematol 57:61–70
6. Dacie JV and Lewis SM (1975) Basic haematological Techniques in practical Haematology, 5th edition. Longman group Ltd, pp 21–67
7. Durate L, Lopez-Sandeval R, Esquiral F and Sanchez-Medal L (1972) Androstane therapy of aplastic anaemia. Acta Hematol (Basel) 47:140–145
8. Fliedner TM, Calvo W, Grilli G (1980) Fetal liver: A transitory site for haematopoietic stem cells replication and selective differentiation. In: Lucarelli G, Fliedner TM, Gale RP (eds) Fetal Liver Transplantation. Current Concepts and future Directions. Amsterdam: Excerpta Medica, pp 5–13

9. Gale RP (1979) Aplastic anaemia: Treatment with anabolic steroids. Br J Haematol 43:483

10. Gale RP, Champlin RE, Feig SA, Fitchen JH (1981) Aplastic anemia: Biology and treatment. Ann Int Med 95:477–494

11. Gale RP (1980) Concepts of fetal liver transplantation in man. In: Lucarelli G, Fliedner TM, Gale RP (eds) Fetal Liver Transplantation. Current Concepts and future Directions. Amsterdam: Excerpta Medica, pp 247–256

12. Kansal V, Sood SK, Batra AK, Adhar G, Malayiya AK, Kucheria K and Balakrishnan K (1979) Fetal liver transplantation in aplastic anemia. Acta Haematol 62:128–136

13. Kansal V (1981) Fetal liver transplantation in aplastic anemia. (Sys Lecture). J Soc Young Scientists 2:8–9

14. Kelemen E (1973) Recovery from chronic idiopathic bone marrow aplasia of young mother after intravenous injection of unprocessed cells from the liver (and Yolk Sac) of her 22 mm. CR-length embryo. Scand J Haemat 10:305–308

15. Kochupillai V, Sharma S, Sundaram KR (1984) Anabolic steroids in aplastic anemia. Ind J Med Res. 80:174–179

16. Kochupillai V, Sharma S, Francis S, Mehra NK, Nanu A, Kalra V, Menon PSN, Bhargava M (1985) Bone marrow reconstiution following human fetal liver infusion (FLI) in sixteen severe aplastic anemia patients. In: Gale RP, Touraine JL, Lucarelli G (eds) Fetal liver transplantation. New York: Alan R Liss, pp 251–265

17. Kochupillai V (1984) Management of aplastic anemia. Ind J Hematol 3:149–154

18. Kubanek B, Rencricca N, Porcellini A, Howard D, Stohlman F (1969) The pattern of recovery of erythropoiesis in heavily irradiated mice receiving transplant of fetal liver. Proc Soc Exp Biol Med 131:831–834

19. Lowenberg B (1980) Lymphocyte maturation and graft vs host disease following fetal liver transplantation. In: Lucarelli G. Fliedner TM, Gale RP (eds) Fetal Liver Transplantation. Current Concepts and future Directions. Amsterdam: Excerpta Medica pp 198–202

20. Lynch RE, Williams DM, Reading JC, Cartright GE (1975) The prognosis in aplastic anemia. Blood 45:517–528

21. Lucarelli G, Izzi T, Porcellini A, Delfini C, Polchi P, Moretti L, Manna A, Grilli G (1980) Fetal liver transplantation in aplastic anemia and acute leukemia. In: Lucarelli G, Fliedner TM, Gale RP (eds) Fetal Liver Transplantation. Current Concepts and future Directions. Amsterdam: Excerpta Medica, pp 284–299

22. Mehra NK, Taneja V, Jhingan B, Sharma S, Kochupillai V: HLA status following fetal liver infusion in aplastic anemia and acute myeloid leukemia. Thymus (this issue)

23. Najeen Y (1981) Long term followup in patients with aplastic anemia. A study of 137 androgen treated patients, surviving more than two years. Am J Med 71:543–551

24. Nissen C, Cornu P, Gratwohl A, Speck B (1980) Antilymphocyte globulin vs bone marrow transplantation in the treatment of severe aplastic anemia. In: Lucarelli G, Fliedner TM, Gale RP (eds) Fetal liver transplantation. Current Concepts and future Directions. Amsterdam: Excerpta Medica, pp 230–236

25. O'Reilly RJ, Phawa R, Kanan W, Kapoor M, Sorell M, Meyers P, Good RA (1977) Reconstitution of hematopoietic function in posthepatic aplasia following high dose cyclophosphamide and allogeneic fetal liver transplantation. Exp Hematol 5(suppl 2):46

26. Sanchez-Medal L, Gomez-Leal A, Durate L, Gyadalupe Rico M (1969) Anabolic androgenic steroids in the treatment of acquired aplastic anemia. Blood 34:283–300

27. Shadduck RK, Pigoli G, Waheed A, Bolgal F (1980) Characterization of hemopoietic progenitor cells in fetal liver. In: Lucarelli G, Fliedner TM, Gale RP (eds) Fetal Liver Transplantation. Current Concepts and future Directions. Amsterdam: Excerpta Medica, pp 29–36

28. Scott RB, Malthias JQ, Constrandonlakis M, Key HEM, Lucas PF (1961) Hypoplastic anemia treated by transfusion of fetal hemopoietic cells. Brit Med J 2:1385–1388

29. Sharma S, Bhargava M, Takkar D, Kochupillai V (1985) Morphological pattern of hematopoiesis in human fetal liver. In: Gale RP, Touraine JL, Lucarelli G (eds) Fetal Liver Transplantation. New York: Alan R. Liss, pp 167–171

30. Speck B, Gratwohl A, Nissen C, Ruggaro D, Cornu P, Burri HP, Jeannet M (1980) Severe aplastic anemia: A prospective study on the value of different therapeutic approaches in 37 successive patients. Blut 41:160–163

31. Territt MC for the UCLA Bone marrow transplant team: Autologous bone marrow repopulation following high dose cyclophosphamide and allogeneic bone marrow transplantation in aplastic anemia. Br J Haematol 36:305–312

Thymus 10:103–108 (1987)
© Martinus Nijhoff Publishers, Dordrecht

Bone marrow recovery following fetal liver infusion (FLI) in aplastic anaemia: Morphological studies

M. BHARGAVA,[1] A.K. KARAK,[1] S. SHARMA[2] and V. KOCHUPILLAI[2]

[1] Departments of Pathology (Haematology Unit) and [2] Medical Oncology, All India Institute of Medical Sciences, Ansari Nagar, New Delhi, IND-110029, India

Key words: aplastic anaemia, fetal liver infusion, bone marrow morphology

Summary. Twenty-two of 35 patients with aplastic anaemia who received fetal liver infusion (FLI), responded to this treatment. Detailed review of bone marrow aspirates and biopsies was available in 17. There was a good correlation between clinical improvement and blood counts. The bone marrow cellularity increased to 48 percent in about 18 weeks with repopulation by both erythroid and myeloid cells. The erythroid response was predominant and the earliest to occur (1.5–61 weeks); it lasted for 7.5–100 weeks. Marked dyserythropoiesis was observed. Myeloid response occurred simultaneously in 45 percent of the responders; in the others it was delayed by 1.5 to 4 weeks. Significant dysmyelopoiesis with shift to the left, unrelated to infection, was seen 1.5 to 9.5 weeks after FLI lasting for 9–26 weeks in most cases. Megakaryocytic response either did not occur or was delayed, less marked and often transient.

Introduction

Fetal liver infusion is a relatively new method of treatment of severe aplastic anaemia. There is a paucity of information on bone marrow morphological changes in recipients of fetal liver. A retrospective study was therefore carried out to note in detail the morphological changes in recovering bone marrow following fetal liver infusion.

Material and methods

A total of 40 patients with severe aplastic anaemia received fetal liver infusion 1 to 4 times during the course of their disease. Their follow-up ranged between 1.8 to 100 months. Thirty-five patients were evaluable and, of these, 22 responded (62%). In 17 patients, a review of peripheral blood counts, bone marrow aspirates and bone biopsies was available. There were 16 males and 1 female, ranging in age from 10 to 70 years. History of ingestion of analgesics in 3 and of chloramphenicol in 1 was available. Eleven were idiopathic and 2 had pure red cell aplasia.

Address for offprints: Dr. Manorama Bhargava, Associate Professor, Haematology Unit, Department of Pathology, All India Institute of Medical Sciences, Ansari Nagar, New Delhi, IND-110029, India.

Table 1. Haemoglobin, absolute granulocyte count and platelet count in 17 patients with aplastic anaemia following fetal liver infusion.

Serial number	Haemoglobin (g/dl)	Absolute granulocyte count (per mm^3)	Platelet count ($\times 10^3$ per mm^3)
1	13.9	2916	90
2	12.3	2320	80
3	8.0	1584	50
4	6.0	578	70
5[a]	6.0	2040	40
6	11.8	2928	180
7	9.5	1900	46
8[a]	6.7	5285	160
9	13.2	2016	87
10	12.3	2652	110
11	7.8	1008	40
12	11.4	3240	110
13	10.2	3200	90
14	8.0	1615	100
15	8.5	1590	40
16	8.2	1750	40
17	6.5	1404	90

[a] Two patients with pure red cell aplasia in whom the response was judged by increase in haemoglobin alone.

The bone marrows were reviewed by two of us (M.B. and A.K.) without prior information on the clinical data. The bone marrow cellularity was assessed according to Hartsock et al. [3].

Results

Table 1 shows the values of haemoglobin, absolute granulocyte count and the platelet count following fetal liver infusion. According to the criteria defined elsewhere [6], the improvement in these blood counts from the pre-fetal liver infusion values justified the following classification: good response in 7, moderate response in 5 and minimal response in 5 patients. The bone marrow cellularity increased in all cases but two and, from virtually empty bone marrows (Figure 1), reached a cellularity of 29 to 86 percent by 18 weeks (Figure 2). The response was slow in all haematologic parameters, taking nearly 16 to 18 weeks to reach a maximum value.

The erythroid response was the most predominant and the first to occur in the bone marrow, with myeloid erythroid ratios of 1:1.6 to 1:5.7. It occurred within 1.5 to 61 weeks of fetal liver infusion (median: 14 weeks) and lasted from 7.5 to 100 weeks (median 51 weeks). There was marked dyserythropoiesis with megaloblastoid changes (Figure 3), budding, rhexis, binucleated cells and giant forms.

In 50 percent of the cases, a myeloid response occurred simultaneously with the erythroid response, but in the remaining 50 percent it occurred 1.5 to 4 weeks later. In a majority of patients (11/17), it lasted as long as the

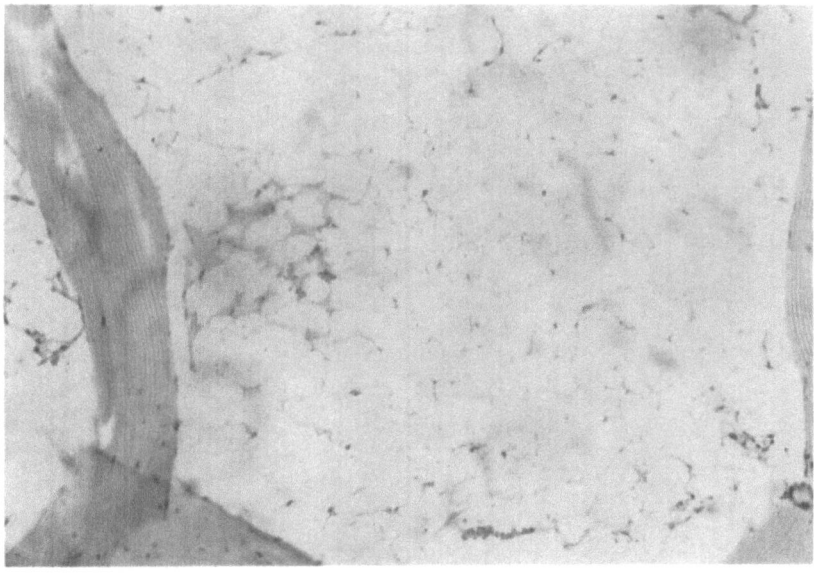

Figure 1. Bone marrow biopsy from a patient with severe aplastic anaemia before FLI, showing marked hypocellularity. (Hematoxylin — Eosin. × 75.)

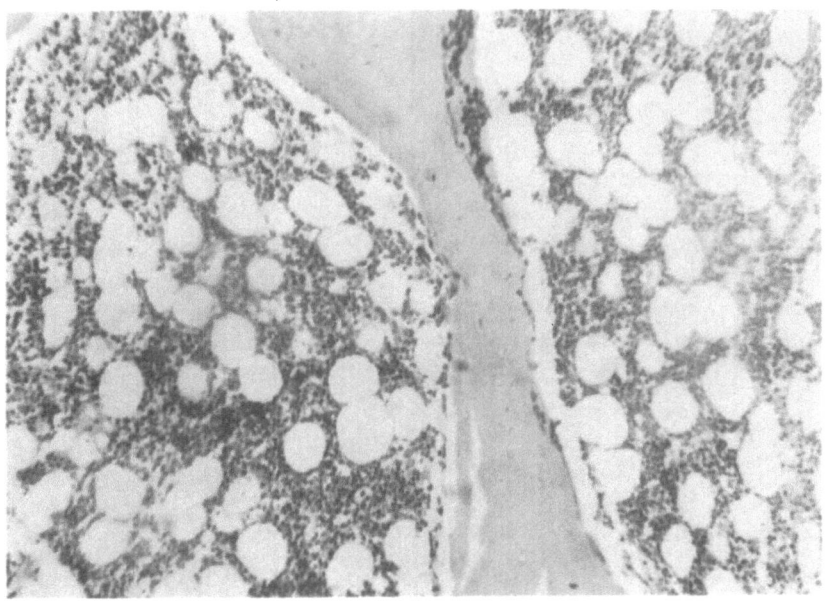

Figure 2. Bone marrow biopsy from the same patient as in Figure 1, 14 weeks after FLI, showing markedly increased cellularity. (Hematoxylin — × 75.)

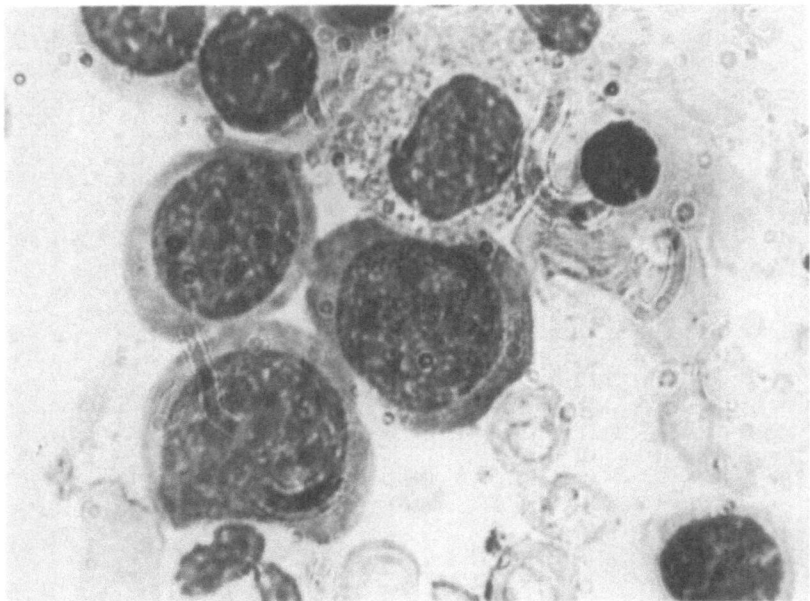

Figure 3. Bone marrow aspirate, 14 weeks following FLI, showing pronounced megaloblastoid change in the erythroid precursors. (Jenner — Giemsa. × 750.)

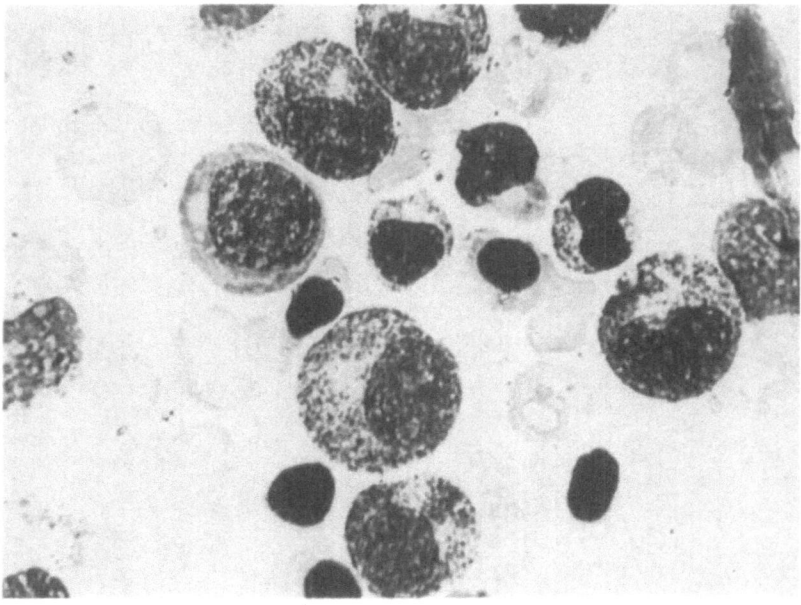

Figure 4. Bone marrow aspirate, 14 weeks following FLI, showing dysmyelopoiesis with hypergranulation. (Jenner — Giemsa. × 750.)

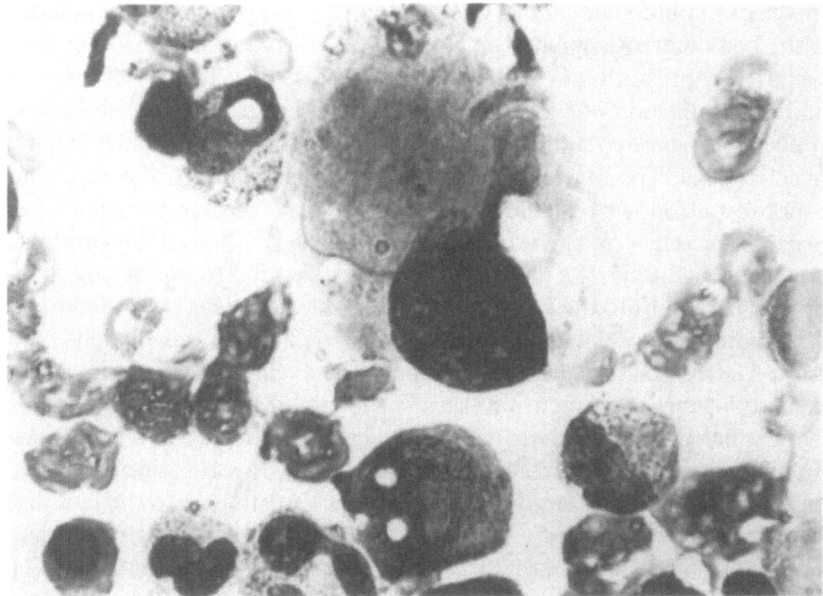

Figure 5. Bone marrow aspirate, 14 weeks following FLI, showing mononuclear megakaryocyte with no evidence of platelet formation. (Jenner — Giemsa. × 750.)

erythroid response but in 5 of the 17 cases, the duration was shorter by 4 to 13 weeks. There was evidence of dysmyelopoiesis with hypergranulation (Figure 4), hypogranulation and pseudo-Pelger anomaly. Pronounced shift to the left occurred within 1.5 to 9 weeks of fetal liver infusion and was persistent in about half the cases; in the other half, it subsided in about 19 weeks. Shift to the left had no relationship with infection.

Megakaryocytic response usually did not occur. When it did, it was minimal, with hypodiploid or mononuclear forms (Figure 5).

In all instances, the bone marrow lymphocyte count decreased to less than 10 percent following fetal liver infusion.

Discussion

A definite improvement in haemoglobin, total leucocyte and absolute granulocyte count with concomitant with clinical improvement occurs following fetal liver infusion in patients with severe aplastic anaemia. In some patients, repeated fetal liver infusions are necessary to sustain improvement. The effect on platelets is slower and only marginal. Beneficial effects of FLI in severe aplastic anaemia have been reported by other workers as well [4, 5, 7].

To our knowledge, there is as yet no information available on bone marrow changes following fetal liver infusion. In our patients, the improvement in blood counts was associated with a significant repopulation of the bone marrow by both myeloid and erythroid cells, predominantly the latter, contributing to a considerable increase in cellularity of the post fetal liver infusion bone marrow. The erythroid response was the earliest to occur; it persisted and outlasted the myeloid response, sometimes by several weeks. The myeloid response occurred either with the erythroid response or followed it and was generally of a shorter duration. The megakaryocytes were slow to appear, if at all, and showed morphologic atypism. Qualitatively, there was striking dyserythropoiesis, dysmyelopoiesis and shift to the left. In some cases, these changes were so marked as to resemble a preleukaemic state. However, none of our patients who showed such a picture, evolved into acute leukaemia. Besides, consistent haematologic improvement was seen in the face of these dyshaemopoietic changes indicating that these might have been an evidence of a repopulating bone marrow with reconstitution of bone marrow function. A persistent, predominant erythroid response further lent support to the fact that the bone marrow recovery following fetal liver infusion might be associated with an accelerated, albeit partial recapitulation of ontogeny [1]. Similar morphologic changes have been seen following anti-lymphocyte globulin treatment of aplastic anaemia (B. Speck, personal communication). Spontaneous recovery in aplastic anaemia is also associated with disordered haemopoiesis [2]. That fetal liver infusion stimulates bone marrow regenerative activity resulting in haematologic improvement, appears undoubtful but the mechanism of this action is not clear. None of the patients in this group showed evidence of engraftment [6]. A slow and partial recovery, unlike that seen in human bone marrow transplantation, further suggests autologous bone marrow regeneration to an as yet undefined stimulus.

References

1. Alter BP, Rappopport JM, Huisman THJ, Schroeder WA, Nathan DG (1976) Fetal erythropoiesis following bone marrow transplantation. Blood 48:843–853
2. Gordon-Smith EC (1977) Aplastic anaemia: Speculations on pathogenesis. In: Lewis SM and Verwilghen RL (eds) Dyserythropoiesis. London: Academic Press, pp 149–162
3. Hartsock RJ, Smith EB, Petty CS (1965) Normal variations with aging of the amount of hematopoietic tissue in bone marrow from the anterior iliac crest. Am J Clin Path 43:326–331
4. Kansal V, Sood SK, Batra AK, Adhar G, Malviya AK, Kucheria K, Balakrishnan K (1979) Fetal liver transplantation in aplastic anemia. Acta Haematologica 62:128–136
5. Kelemen E (1973) Recovery from chronic idiopathic bone marrow aplasia of a young mother after intravenous injection of unprocessed cells from the liver (and yolk sac) of her 22 mm CR-length embryo. Scand J Haemat 10:305–308
6. Kochupillai V, Sharma S, Francis S, Nanu A, Susan M, Bhatia P, Dua H, Kumar L, Aggarwal S, Singh S, Kumar S, Karak A, Bhargava M: Fetal liver infusion in aplastic anaemia. Thymus (this issue)
7. Scott RB, Matthias JQ, Constandoulakis M, Kay HEM, Lucas PF, Whiteside JD (1961) Hypoplastic anemia treated by transfusion of foetal haemopoietic cells. Brit Med J 2:1385–1388

Thymus 10:109–116 (1987)

Advances in experimental studies and clinical application of fetal liver cells

CHU TSE WU[1] and GEN YAD YE

[1] Department of Experimental Hematology, Institute of Radiation Medicine, P.O. Box 130, Beijing; [2] North Tai-Ping Road Hospital, Beijing, China

Key words: fetal liver transfusion, fetal liver transplantation, ontogenetic barrier, histoincompatibility barrier

Introduction

In 1958, Uphoff [1] reported the effectiveness of fetal liver transplantation in promoting hematopoietic recovery of lethally irradiated mice. In 1959, Thomas et al. [2] attempted fetal liver transfusion in leukemic patients who received radiotherapy. Recently, studies of transplantation of hematopoietic stem cells derived from fetal liver, have been reported in patients with hematological disorders.

Fetal liver transfusion

Respone criteria

Standard criteria for diagnosis of aplastic anemia and evaluation of response have been reported [3]. Two types of aplastic anemia were identifed: (a) acute aplastic anemia characterized by sudden anemia with corrected reticulocytes less than 1%, neutrophils less than $0.5 \times 10^9/l$, platelets less than $10\text{--}20 \times 109/l$ accompanied by serious infection and hemorrhage; (b) chronic aplastic anemia with less serious infection, anemia and hemorrhage.

The following criteria were used to evaluate the effectiveness of treatment: (1) *cure*: hemoglobin $> 12\,g/dl$ for males or $> 10\,g/dl$ for females, WBC $> 4 \times 10^9/l$, platelets $> 80 \times 10^9/l$, no relapse following g > 1 year of observation; (2) *remission*: hemoglobin $> 12\,g/dl$ for males and $> 10\,g/dl$ for females, WBC $> 3.5 \times 10^9/l$, platelets improved, condition is stable or gradually improves within 3 months of observation; (3) *improvement*: no blood transfusion is required; hemoglobin increased by $3\,g/l$ above pretreatment value within 3 months following treatment; or no response. (4) *clinical effectiveness of fetal liver transfusion*: fetal liver transfusion refers to patients receiving transfusions of fetal liver cells without pretransfusion immune suppression.

Lucarelli et al. [4] reported 26 patients with severe aplastic anemia who failed to respond to standard therapy, and who were transfused with fetal liver cells obtained from 3 to 6 months fetuses. Nine patients have an improvement in hematopoiesis within 10–55 days, 5 (19%) recovered normal hemotopoiesis within 2–5 years. Temporary chimera was detected in 3 cases.

In our chinese cooperative group, a considerable number of patients with acute and chronic aplastic anemia have received single or multiple fetal liver transfusions. Short-term improvement was observed in 40%. Lou et al. [5] reported improvement in 36 out of 56 cases (65%) of chronic aplastic anemia following multiple transfusions of fetal liver cells. Four fetal livers were transfused successively in most cases. Seventeen percent of patients were cured. Similar results were observed in 4 cases of acute aplastic anemia. One patient showed short-term improvement; another one has recovered normal hemopoiesis during a course of observation of more than one year and was cured.

Characteristics of patients who respond to fetal liver transfusion are as follows. Reticulocytes are the most sensitive indicator of recovery of hemopoiesis, followed by hemoglobin, WBC and platelets. In responders the requirement of blood transfusion is reduced or discontinued and patients are subjectively improved. In general, multiple transfusions of fetal liver cells result in a higher cure rate. It is possible that the different types of response to fetal liver transfusion may reflect diverse etiologies of aplastic anemia in the patient.

Mechanism of the action of fetal liver transfusion in aplastic anemia

We used chromosome C-banding to analyse the karyotype of peripheral lymphocytes or bone marrow cells in 29 patients with aplastic anemia or leukemia 1–3 months after fetal liver transfusion. No direct evidence of engraftment of transfused fetal liver cells was observed. What is the possible mechanism of fetal liver transfusion in stimulating the recovery of hemopoiesis in aplastic anemia patients? The following are two possibilities:

(a) Stimulation of hemopoiesis

Because of the complex etiology of aplastic anemia Ji et al. [6] adopted a self-comparison method to judge the possible effect of fetal liver transfusion on hematopoiesis. A group of leukemia patients received two similar courses of chemotherapy given one month apart. After the first course of chemotherapy, peripheral blood counts recovered slowly. When a fetal liver cell suspension was transfused after the end of the second course of chemotherapy, recovery of blood counts, including reticulocytes,

WBC and platelets, was markedly accelerated. These data suggest a stimulatory effect of fetal liver cell transfusion on the recovery of hemopoiesis. Other experiments in our laboratory indicate that extracts of fetal liver cells destroyed by ultrasound strongly stimulate erythropoiesis and enhance the phagocytic activity of peritoneal macrophages in normal or plethoric mice [7]. Based on these experimental findings Lei Lun et al. (submitted) used the supernatant of fetal liver cells lysed with hypotonic solution to treat patients with chronic aplastic anemia. Improvement was observed following 20–40 injections of this material. These data indicate that besides the possible temporary engraftment of transfused hematopoietic stem cells from fetal liver, some humoral factor that can stimulate hematopoiesis may be present in fetal liver cells. The biochemical nature of this factor is unknown.

(b). Non specific immune activity

Fetal liver cell transfusions were given to 14 patients with aplastic anemia. Eleven patients showed an increase in erytrhocyte-rosette (E-RFC) and α-napthyl acetate esterase (ANAE) positive cells in peripheral blood (Table 1); no change was observed in 3 cases. The possibility that fetal liver cell transfusion results in a stimulation of non specific immune function has been discussed (Li Chun-hui et al., submitted). Transfusion of allogeneic fetal liver cells, might activate recipient T-lymphocyte. This hypothesis is supported by the observation that giant E-rosette formation is frequently observed in peripheral lymphocytes of patients receiving transfusions of fetal liver cells.

Table 1. Changes of peripheral T-lymphocyte in patients with aplastic anemia following transfusion of fetal liver cell suspension (average ± S.D.).

Time (days)	Number of cases	E-RFC/mm^{3a}	ANAE cells/mm^{3b}
Before trans- fusion	8	385 ± 166	696 ± 250
After trans- fusion			
5	9	1020 ± 289	1420 ± 753
10	8	1250 ± 784	1643 ± 780
15	7	1316 ± 701	1172 ± 390
20	7	983 ± 166	1244 ± 661
25	10	732 ± 298	946 ± 268
30	3	662 ± 294	1435 ± 149
35	2	839 ± 275	1218 ± 448
40	4	596 ± 166	923 ± 16
50	6	955 ± 544	1251 ± 286
62	5	865 ± 335	1192 ± 330

[a] E-rosette formation.
[b] Acid-esterase staining method.

Clinical application of fetal liver cells in the treatment of radiation sickness

After a radiation accident in Yugoslavia [8], a patient was simultaneously transfused with allogeneic fetal liver and bone marrow cells. Evaluation of therapeutic effect is difficult as the cells were given after a long interval. In 1980, a patient was exposed to 5.2 Gy gamma rays in China. He received a fetal liver cell suspension from a 4.5 month old male fetus on day 5 after irradiation. Following this the absolute number of peripheral lymphocytes progressively increased and E-RFC markedly increased in size. The response of T-lymphocytes to PHA was increased. These observations indicate the functional activation of T-lymphocytes following transfusion of fetal liver cells. After irradiation reticulocytes progressively decreased from 0.004% to 0.0009% and remained at this level for 6 to 11 days.

The mitotic index of bone marrow cells markedly increased from 0 to 0.6% after transfusion of fetal liver cells. Erythroblasts were found in bone marrow. This improvement in erythropoiesis may have resulted from temporary engraftment of hemopoietic cells of fetal liver origin or by stimulation of endogenous erythropoiesis by the transfused fetal liver cells. Because the sex of the fetus was identical to the recipient, no direct evidence of engraftment could be obtained. However, the immune and hematologic responses to fetal liver transfusion were similar to those observed in the patients with aplastic anemia or with leukemia after chemotherapy who received fetal liver transfusion [9].

Progress of fetal liver transplantation in leukemia treatment

Touraine [10] reported progress in the therapy of severe combined immunodeficiency diseases with fetal liver transplantation. Since 1978 Izzi and colleagues [11] have transplanted 18 patients with severe aplastic anemia (5 cases) or leukemia (13 cases) with fetal liver cells after preconditioning with high doses of cytotoxic drugs and 10 Gy total body irradiation. In most cases temporary engraftment was observed. Interestingly, one case of long term chimera (up to 240 days after transplantation) was reported.

Since 1980, clinical studies of fetal liver transplantation have developed rapidly in China. Presently, 12 patients including 10 with acute leukemia and 2 with B-thalassemia major have received fetal liver transplants [12–14]. Pretransplant conditioning included high doses of cyclophosphamide (80 mg/kg) and total body irradiation (5.5–7 Gy). Either a single or multiple fetal livers were transfused successively within one week following irradiation. Only a small number of chimeras could be detected within 30–50 days after transplantation in most instances. One patient transplanted with a fetal liver from a fetus of opposite sex had substantial numbers of donor cells up to 300 days post-transplant. Then progressively decreased from 85% to 40% on day 240 (Liu Yong-xing et al., submitted).

Table 2. Results of fetal liver transplantation in the patients after preconditioning with cyclophosphamide (Cy) and total body irradiation (TBI).

| Patient | | | preconditioning | Fetus | | Result | | survival time post FLT | outcome |
case	age sex	diagnosis status		number	sex	engraftment	GVHD		
1	13 m	ALL/1	Cy + TBI	1	1 f	Day 30 10%(XX)[a]	no	+360	relapse
2	6 f	ALL/1	Cy + TBI	1	1 m	no	no	>810	CR
3	9 m	AGL/1	Cy + TBI	1	1 m	yes[b]	no	+205	relapse
4	7 m	ALL/3	Cy + DNR + TBI	5	3 f, 2 m	Day 30 3%(XX)	no	+135	relapse
5	12 m	ALL/1	Cy + DNR + TBI	6	3 f, 3 m	Day 15 2%(XX)	no	>800	CR
6	21 m	AMo/1	Cy + Ara – C + TBI	8	5 f, 3 m	Day 30 5%(XX)	mild	>560	CR
7	10 m	APML/1	Cy + DNR + TBI	5	3 f, 2 m	no	no	>430	CR
8	20 m	ALL/1	Cy + DNR + TBI	5	3 f, 2 m	Day 15 70%(XX)	no	+60	IP
9	22 m	AML/1	Cy + TBI	11	4 f, 7 m	Day 30 5%(XX)	no	>150	CR
10	18 m	ALL/1	Cy + TBI	5	5 f	Day 30 60%(XX) Day 147 70%(XX)	mild	>330	CR
11	4 f	Thalassemia	Cy + TBI	4	2 m, 2 f	Day 30 80%(XX) Day 150 0%(XY)	mild	>240	improvement
12	2 m	Thalassemia	Cy + TBI	3	2 m, 1 f	Day 30 20%(XX) Day 60 0%(XX)	no	>240	CR

[a] % of donor karyotype in bone marrow or peripheral blood.
[b] Red cell isoenzyme determination   DNR: Daunoruoicin   m: male   f: female   CR: complete remission

In most cases of fetal liver transplantation no symptoms of GVHD or only mild GVHD was observed. Among the 10 leukemia patients, 6 survived 135 to 810 days post-transplant; two have survived more than 800 days (Table 2).

Ontogenetic and histoincompatibility barriers to allogeneic fetal liver transplantation

During gestation, hematopoietic stem cells migrate from the yolk sac to the liver and bone marrow. This may be accompanied by changes in the morphology and other properties of these cells.

A group of LACA mice was irradiated (8.0 Gy) and transplanted with 9×10^6 fetal liver cells and 3×10^6 adult bone marrow cells, both containing approximately the same number of CFU-S. We used female mice as recipients and normal male mice as donors of the bone marrow. Fetal liver cells were taken from embryos of both sexes because the sex difference was indistinguishable at this early gestational age. We assumed that fetal liver cells prepared from 20 fetuses in this experiment had an equal chance of being male or female. C-banding techniques were used to identify the sex of bone marrow or fetal liver cells taken from recipients after transplantation. The purpose of this experiment was to determine the competition of hemopoietic stem cells from either source in reestablishing hemopoiesis in lethally irradiated mice. Twenty days after transplantation there were only 7.9% with female chromosome cells in the recipient bone marrow. This is less than the theoritical value of 25%. Thereafter, the proportion of cells in bone marrow with a female karyotype increased gradually, reaching 49% on day 62 (Figure 1). This indicates that nearly all cells in recipient bone marrow were finally replaced by the cells of fetal liver origin. These data suggest that hemopoietic stem cells from the murine fetal liver have a lower seeding efficiency than adult bone marrow cells on day 20. In adult recipients, after a short period of delay, the ability of self-renewal and proliferation of fetal liver cells was greatly enhanced compared to that of bone marrow [15]. This is consistent with the results of competitive proliferation of fetal and adult hemopoietic cells in lethally irradiated mice using the T6 chromosome marker [16].

In the experiments described, recipients and donors were inbred LACA mice. Therefore, the lower seeding efficiency of hemopoietic stem cells from fetal liver in adult spleen or bone marrow can not be attributed to histoincompatibility, and is more likely related to different stages of ontogenetic development. This may affect the migration of immature CFU-S from fetal liver to adult bone marrow. Adult bone marrow is assumed to have spacial structures called 'niches' which accommodate hemopoietic stem cells. These 'niches' may only be suitable for stem cells destined to migrate to the bone marrrow but not for cells destined to

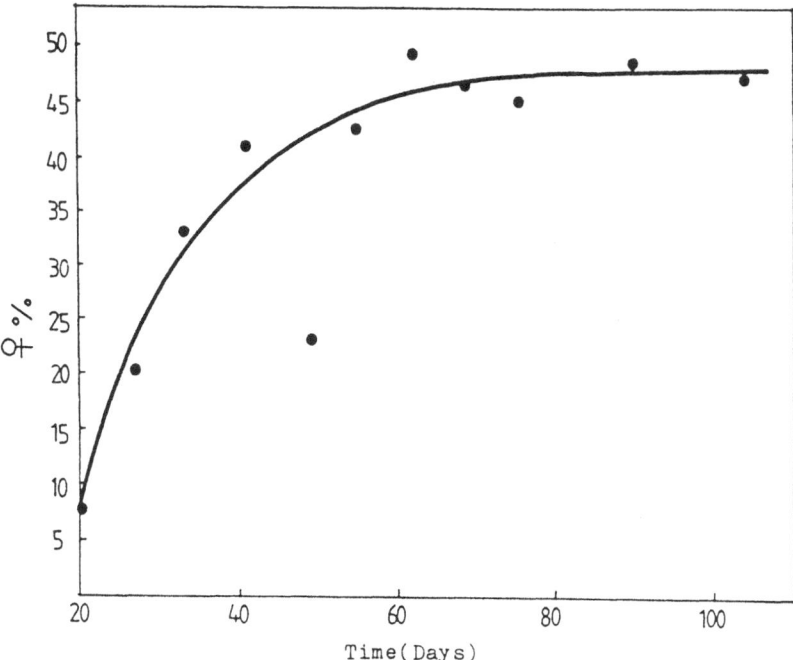

Figure 1. Kinetic changes of cells with female sex chromosome in the bone marrow of irradiated recipient mice after transfusion of a mixture of normal bone marrow and fetal liver cells containing equal numbers of CFU-S.

migrate to fetal liver. This may explain the observation that fetal liver cells are more difficult to engraft in adult hemopoietic organs.

Short-term, in vitro culture may alter some peculiarities of hemopoietic stem cells of fetal liver origin. This might reduce the aforementioned ontogenetic barrier and improve the seeding efficiency or adaptibility of fetal liver derived hemopoietic stem cells. Our preliminary experiments show that fetal liver cells cultured for 6-days in diffusion chamber in vivo have an increase of seeding efficiency in the spleen and bone marrow of 8.0 Gy irradiated adult syngeneic mice.

Besides an ontogenetic barrier, there is also an allogeneic transplantation resistence due to histocompatibility between donor and recipient. Animal experiments consistently demonstrate that the degree of allogeneic transplantation resistance can be greatly ameliorated by high doses of immunosuppressors. Short-term culture of fetal liver cells in diffusion chambers increases seeding efficiency of FLT in adult hemopoietic organs, in syngeneic but not allogeneic conditions. From these experimental results, it seems likely that a histoincompatible barrier plays a more important role than an ontogenetic barrier in allogeneic fetal liver transplantation [17].

116

References

1. Uphoff DE: Preclusion of secondary phase of irradiation syndrome by inoculation of fetal hemopoietic tissue following lethal total-body X-irradiation. J Nat Cancer Inst 20: 625, 1958
2. Thomas ED, Lochte HL Jr., Ferrebee JW: Irradiation of the entire body and marrow transplantation: Some observation and comments Blood 14: 1, 1959
3. Proceedings on etiology, diagnosis, typing and treatment of aplastic anemia. Chinese J Hemat 2: 199, 1981
4. Lucarelli G, Izzi T, Porcellini A et al.: Fetal Liver Transplantation in aplastic anemia and acute leukemia. In: RP Gale (eds) Recent advances in bone marrow transplantation, AR Liss, New York, 1983, p 865
5. Lou FD, Liu HC, Wang YZ: Short-term and multiole fetal liver transplantation (FLT) for treatment of aplastic anemia: Report of 15 cases. Chinese J Inter Med 24: 65, 1985
6. Ji SQ, Zhu M, Ke ZM et al.: The effectiveness of fetal liver transfusion in the treatment of aplastic anemia and leukemia after chemotherapy. Beijing Medical Journal 6: 6, 1984
7. Wu CT, Chen JP, Xue HH, Tian HB, Zhou SZ, Liu XY: Studies on the mechanism of fetal liver transfusion or whole embryonic extract injection in the treatment of aplastic anemia. Chinese J. Applied Physiol 1: 9, 1985
8. Жаммэ А, Матэ Г, Латаржэи Р: Шестб случаев острой лучевой болезии у пострадавщих при аварии ядерного реактора в югославии. Мед. Радиол. 4(9): 83, 1959
9. Yie GY, Qian FW, Mao BZ, et al.: Instructors: Tian N, Wu CT: A case of severe hemopoietic form of radiation sickness. Chinese J. Med. 1986 (in press).
10. Touraine JL: Fetal and thymus transplantation in immunodeficiencies and inborn errors of metabolism: medical, immunological and ethical aspects. Second International Symposium on Fetal Liver Transplantation (Abstract) 1984, 19
11. Izzi T, Polchi P, Galimberti M, et al.: Fetal Liver Transplantation in aplastic anemia and acute leukemia. In: Riss AR (ed) Fetal Liver Transplantation, New York, 1985, pp 237–249
12. Meng PL, Fei RG, Gu DW: Allogeneic fetal liver transplantation in acute leukemia. In: AR Riss (ed) Fetal Liver Transplantation, New York, 1985, pp 281–291
13. Yao SQ, Liu HC, Lou FD et al.: Fetal liver transplants in the treatment of adult Amol. A case report. Med J Chinese PLA 10(5): 339, 1985
14. Liu HC: Allogeneic fetal liver transplantation in the treatment of acute leukemia. Report of 5 cases. Chinese J Hemat 1986 (in press)
15. Wu CT, Zhang YH: Peculiarities of hemopoietic stem cell transplantation from fetal liver. Acta Physiologica Sinica 36 (1): 70, 1984
16. Micklem HS, Ford CE, Evans EP, et al.: Competitive in vivo proliferation of fetal and adult haemopoietic cells in lethally irradiated mice. J Cell Physiol 79: 293, 1972
17. Wu CT: Experimental studies on hemopoietic stem cells of fetal liver origin and its clinical application. In: AR Liss (ed), Fetal Liver Transplantation, New York, 1985, pp 95–112

Thymus 10:117–124 (1987)
© Martinus Nijhoff Publishers, Dordrecht

Fetal liver infusion in acute myelogenous leukaemia

V. KOCHUPILLAI, S. SHARMA, S. FRANCIS, A. NANU,[1] I.C. VERMA,[2] H. DUA,
L. KUMAR, S. AGGARWAL and S. SINGH

Medical Oncology Department, Institute Rotary Cancer Hospital, [1] Blood Bank,
[2] Paediatric Department, All India Institute of Medical Sciences, New Delhi, India

Key words: fetal liver infusion, transient engraftment, acute myeloid leukaemia

Summary. Forty-five patients with acute myelogenous leukaemia (AML) received induction chemotherapy with either a conventional dose of cytarabine and daunorubicin (27 patients) or a low dose of cytarabine (18 patients). Maintenance chemotherapy was given to all responders. In 14 of 39 evaluable patients, infusion of fetal liver cells from 10–24 weeks old foetuses was given following induction as well as maintenance therapy. Six of 14 patients (43%) achieved a complete remission; 2 showed evidence of transient engraftment documented by analysis of sex chromosomes and RBC antigens (1 patient each). Fetal liver infusion within 6 days of completing induction chemotherapy appeared more effective than when given later. Five of 25 patients (20%) who did not receive fetal liver infusion achieved a complete remission. The present work suggests that fetal liver infusion given following induction chemotherapy may increase the remission rate in AML either by temporary engraftment or by accelerating the rate of haematological recovery.

Introduction

The intensive chemotherapy used in acute myelogenous leukaemia (AML) is associated with severe bone marrow suppression which can be fatal unless accompanied by effective supportive care [3, 9, 10, 12, 16]. With recent therapy 60–80% of patients achieve complete remission. Median remission duration is 12 to 18 months with 20 to 30% leukaemia free survival of 3–5 years. Most patients relapse, however, and their survival is correspondingly brief [2, 10]. These problems have led to efforts to investigate other modes of treatment for AML including immunotherapy [14], low dose cytarabine [5, 6, 15] and bone marrow transplantation [11, 13]. We describe a novel modality, fetal liver infusion as an adjuvant to study was to determine if the infusion of fetal liver cells was capable of influencing the likelihood of achieving remission in AML and if fetal liver cells would engraft under these conditions.

Address for offprints: Dr. Vinod Kochupillai, Associate Professor of Medical Oncology, Institute Rotary Cancer Hospital, All India Institute of Medical Sciences, New Delhi, IND-110 029, India.

Intensive induction chemotherapy

From April 1982, till November 1984, 27 consecutive previously untreated patients with AML received a combination of daunorubicin $45\,mg/m^2$ intravenously on days 1, 2 and 3, and cytarabine $100\,mg/m^2$ by continuous infusion for 7 days. Peripheral blood counts were determined daily and cytarabine was discontinued if the WBC was less than $10^9/l$. This was necessary in view of limited availability of blood components and antibiotics.

In 12 patients, this chemotherapy could be supplemented by fetal liver infusion within 8 days of the last dose of chemotherapy. With the exception of 2 patients, who received 2 courses of induction chemotherapy at the interval of 1 month, all others received only one course of chemotherapy followed by fetal liver infusion.

Six patients refused fetal liver infusion and, for 9 others, it was not available within 8 days of completing chemotherapy. These 15 patients who did not receive fetal liver cells are considered as the control group; 10 received 1 course and 5 received 2 courses of induction chemotherapy.

Low-dose cytarabine induction therapy

Intensive induction chemotherapy was associated with significant mortality [9, 12]. From December 1984, till November 1985, therefore, 18 consecutive patients received low-dose cytarabine $(10\,mg/m^2)$ every 12 hours subcutaneously for 3 weeks. In 4 patients, of which 2 received one course and 2 received 2 courses, this chemotherapy could be supplemented by fetal liver infusion within 6 days of the last dose of chemotherapy.

In 14 patients, of which 6 received one course and 8 received 2 courses, no fetal liver cells were available within 6 days of completing chemotherapy.

Supportive therapy as described earlier [9] was provided to all patients if and when necessary and available.

Maintenance therapy

Patients who achieved remission after one or two courses of induction therapy received cyclical maintenance chemotherapy (Table 1), as outpatients. Fetal liver infusion was repeated when available during maintenance therapy in those patients who received it during induction therapy (Tables 2 & 3).

Fetal liver infusion

Fifty-seven abortuses were available: 38 following hysterotomy, 10 following prostaglandin injection, 1 after syntocinon drip, 2 after extra-amniotic

Table 1. Maintenance chemotherapy.

Drug	Dose	Days	Method of administration
1st Month			
Cytarabine	100 mg/m^2	1–5	S.C. or I.V.
Daunorubicin	60 mg/m^2	1	I.V.
2nd Month			
Cytarabine	100 mg/m^2	1–5	S.C. or I.V.
6-MP	100 mg/m^2	1–5	Orally
3rd Month			
Cytarabine	100 mg/m^2	1–5	S.C. or I.V.
Vincristine	2 mg	1	I.V.
Prednisolone	40 mg/m^2	1–5	Orally

S.C.: Subcutaneously.
I.V.: Intravenously.

emcradyl injection and 6 after spontaneous abortion. Fetal age deter-mined from the last date of menstruation varied between 10–24 weeks with a median (m) of 17 weeks. Fetal liver cell suspension was prepared as described [8], preserved at 4 °C and given within 1 hour to 18 days (m = 9h). The total fetal liver cell number in each infusion varied bet-ween 0.07 to 39 × 10^8. The number of fetal liver cells given to each patient as well as other information on fetal liver cells, including cell viability, are shown in Tables 2 & 3.

Studies for evidence of engraftment

Details of the study conducted to assess engraftment following fetal liver infusion are described in another paper in this issue [1]. These studies included bone marrow cultures for chromosome analysis, HLA A, B and C typing, RBC typing, and determination of the level of alpha-fetoprotein.

Results

Intensive chemotherapy

Of the 12 patients who received fetal liver cells, 2 died within 5 days of fetal liver infusion and are excluded from further analysis. Of the remaining 10 patients, 5 responded (50%); 4 achieved complete remission (CR) with a median survival (MS) of 24 months and one achieved partial remission (PR) with 3 months survival. Of the 15 patients in the control group, 4 responded (27%); 2 achieved CR with an MS of 19.5 months and 2 achieved PR and died within 4 months.

Low-dose cytarabine induction therapy

Of the 14 patients who did not receive fetal liver infusion, 3 died within 9 days of initiating therapy and one patient stopped therapy on his own on the 10th day; these 4 patients are excluded from further analysis. Of the

Table 2. Fetal liver infusion (FLI) following intensive induction chemotherapy.

Patient No.	Interval between the last dose of 1st induction and FLI (days)	Subsequent chemotherapy (CT) & FLI	Total dose of FLI (×10⁹ cells)	Fetal age (weeks)	Interval between abortion & FLI (hours)	FLI viability (%)	Chimerism (evidence)	Survival time (months)
1	2	17 CT + 11 FLI	5.26	12–24	2–170	70–99	Yes (sex chromosome)	28
2	2	–	0.14	16	2	75	NI	2
3	2	15 CT + 12 FLI	6.9	10–22	1.5–432	90–98	Yes (red cell antigens)	20
4	6	29 CT + 10 FLI	7.6	14–23	3–148	55–99	NI	32
5	4	–	0.078	12	5	65	NI	1
6	1	1 CT + No FLI	0.82	20	4	95	NI	3
7	8	–	0.11	14	1	95	NI	0.6
8	6	1 CT + 1 FLI	0.28	12–16	2–2	95–98	NI	2.5
9	8	–	0.19	18	2	95	NI	0.5
10	1	–	3.9	22	32	90	NI	0.5
11	2	16 CT + 3 FLI	2.2	16–22	8–98	95–99	NI	15.5
12	8	1 CT + No FLI	0.42	17	3	95	NI	1.5

NI: Not identified.

Table 3. Fetal liver infusion (FLI) following low-dose cytarabine.

Patient No.	Interval between the last dose of 1st induction and FLI (days)	Subsequent chemotherapy (CT) and FLI	Total dose of FLI ($\times 10^9$ cells)	Fetal age (weeks)	Interval between abortion & FLI (hours)	FLI viability (%)	Chimerism (evidence)	Survival time (months)
1	4	13 CT + 3 FLI	2.7	14–19	6–148	90–98	NI	14+
2	6	1 CT + No FLI	0.04	19	26.5	98	NI	1.2
3	3	6 CT + 2 FLI	1.2	14–18	6–12	95–98	NI	8
4	2	–	1.3	22	13	98	NI	0.8

NI: Not identified.

remaining 10 patients, 3 achieved CR with an MS of 14 months. Of the 4 patients who received fetal liver cells after chemotherapy, 2 achieved CR with an MS of 11 months.

Assessment of engraftment

One male patient who received fetal liver cells from a female donor showed evidence of temporary engraftment. Another patient who was Rh negative prior to the fetal liver infusion became Rh positive temporarily after fetal liver infusion [1].

Discussion

Intensive chemotherapy (3 days daunorubicin, 7 days cytarabine) in AML is reported to induce remission rates exceeding 70% by some authors [3, 10, 16]. Such a therapy, however, induces severe bone marrow aplasia which may last for several weeks, and aggressive supportive therapy in the form of potent antibiotics and blood component therapy is required to enable the patient to survive this period of aplasia. Availability of such supportive therapy is limited in most centres in India. Combination of daunorubicin and cytarabine therefore, produced significant mortality and only 27% could achieve remission [9 and present communication].

There have been recent reports that low-dose cytarabine may not produce bone marrow aplasia. Instead, it may allow differentiation and induction of blasts to mature into normal cells. The results in AML therapy with low-dose cytarabine have been variable [5, 6, 15]. In one study all 3 patients of AML achieved CR [5], in another 7 out of 9 [6] and in a recent study only 2 patients out of a total of 22 achieved CR [15]. In the present study, 3 patients out of 10 (control group) achieved CR. Addition of fetal liver cells appears to have accelerated the rate of haematologic recovery in both groups (intensive chemotherapy as well as low-dose cytarabine) and remission rate has improved to 50%. However, because of the overall small number in each category this difference is not statistically significant.

The present work demonstrates that following intensive chemotherapy which apparently suppresses the patient's own stem cells temporarily, fetal liver cells are capable of complete engraftment in an adult environment. Patient 1 demonstrated XX chromosomes 4 weeks after the infusion of female fetal liver cells, which was performed following intensive induction therapy; bone marrow chromosomes, however, reverted back to XY pattern, once engrafted cells were rejected. During maintenance therapy and following low-dose cytarabine and fetal liver infusion, engraftment by fetal liver cells did not occur detectably in any patient. It may be postulated that fetal liver cells can induce complete engraftment only if most stem cells are completely suppressed. However, if they are partially suppressed, the fetal liver cells may not produce detectable engraftment. Engraftment by fetal liver cells following intensive induction therapy in AML has been reported by others [4].

The time interval between the last dose of induction chemotherapy and the fetal liver infusion may be important; seven patients could be given fetal liver infusion within 48 hours of the last dose of chemotherapy, 4 of whom responded (3 CR, 1PR). Of the 6 who received fetal liver infusion after 48 hours but in less than 6 days of the last dose of chemotherapy 3 achieved CR, while of those 3 patients who received fetal liver infusion on the 8th day, none achieved remission. Fetal liver cell viability may also be important. Two patients who received fetal liver cells with cell viability of less than 75% during induction therapy failed to achieve remission.

The present work suggests that fetal liver infusion may increase the likelihood of achieving remission in AML. The most plausible explanation is that fetal liver infusion following chemotherapy may decrease the interval of aplasia and thereby decrease the risk of death from infections or bleeding. This is of relevance in developing countries like India where such deaths are difficult to prevent due to the lack of supporting facilities. Shortening of the aplastic period by fetal liver infusion may be due either to temporary engraftment of fetal liver cells or to accelerated recovery of patients' own haematopoietic stem cells.

Acknowledgements

We are thankful to the Department of Science and Technology, Government of India for financing this work and to Dr R.P. Gale, Associate Professor of Medicine at the University of California in Los Angeles, USA, for his valuable suggestions in the preparation of this manuscript. Miss Vandana typed the manuscript.

References

1. Bhatia P, Mathew S, Mehra NK, Jayasuryan N, Sharma S, Francis S, Kochupillai V: Studies on engraftment following fetal liver infusion. Thymus (this issue)
2. Foon KA, Gale RP (1982) Controversies in the therapy of acute myelogenous leukaemia. Am J Med 72:963–979
3. Gale RP, Foon KA, Cline MJ, Zighelboim J (1981) Intensive chemotherapy for acute myelogenous leukaemia. Ann Intern Med 94:753–757
4. Gale RP (1985) Fetal liver transplantation in hematologic disorders. In: Gale RP, Touraine JL, Lucarelli G (eds) Fetal Liver Transplantation. New York: Alan R Liss, pp 293–297
5. Housset M, Daniel M, Degos T (1982) Small doses of Ara-C in the treatment of acute myeloid leukaemia cells. Br J Hematol 51:125–129
6. Ishikora H, Sawada H, Okazaki T, Mochizuki T, Isumi Y, Yamagishi, Morihisa, Uchino H (1984) The effects of low dose Ara-C in acute non-lymphoblastic leukaemias and atypical leukaemia. Br J Hematol 58:9–18
7. Kansal V, Sood SK, Batra AK, Adhar G, Malaviya AK, Kucheria K, Balakrishnan K (1979) Fetal liver transplantation in aplastic anemia. Acta Haematol 62:128–136

8. Kochupillai V, Sharma S, Francis S, Mehra NK, Nanu A, Kalra V, Menon PSN, Bhargava M (1985) Bone Marrow reconstitution following human fetal liver infusion (FLI) in sixteen severe aplastic anemia patients. In: Gale RP, Touraine JL, Lucarelli G (eds) Fetal Liver Transplantation. New York: Alan R Liss, pp 251–265

9. Kochupillai V, Sharma S, Francis S, Mehra NK, Nanu A, Verma IC, Takkar D, Kumar S, Gokhale U (1985) Fetal liver infusion: an adjuvant in the therapy of acute myeloid leukaemia (AML). In: Gale RP, Touraine JL, Lucarelli G (eds) Fetal Liver Transplantation. New York: Alan R Liss, p 267–279

10. Lister TA, Rohatiner A (1984) The management of acute myeloid leukaemia. In: Goldman JM, Preisler H (eds) Leukaemia. London: The Butterworths, pp 136–162

11. O'Reilly RJ (1983) Allogeneic bone marrow transplantation: Current status and future directions. Blood 62:941–964

12. Raina V, Kochupillai V (1983) Acute myeloid leukaemia in adults: Experience at AIIMS. J Assoc Phy Ind 31:511–514

13. Thomas ED, Buckner CD, Cliff RA, Fefer A, Johnson FL, Neiman PE (1979) Marrow transplantation for acute non-lymphoblastic leukaemia in first remission. N Eng J Med 301:597–599

14. Whittaker JA, Bailey-wood R, Hutchins S (1980) Active immunotherapy for the treatment of acute myelogenous leukaemia: Report of two controlled trials. Br J Hematol 45:399–400

15. Winter JN, Variakosis D, Gaynor ER, Larson RA, Miller KB (1985) Low dose cytosine arabinoside (Ara-C) therapy in the myelodysplastic syndromes and acute leukaemia. Cancer 56:443–449

16. Zighelboim J, Foon KA, Gale RP, Haskell CM (1985) Acute myelogenous leukaemia. In: Haskell CM (ed) Cancer Treatment, Second Ed. New York: Saunders WB, p 694

Thymus 10:125–130 (1987)
© Martinus Nijhoff Publishers, Dordrecht

Studies on engraftment following fetal liver infusion

P. BHATIA,[1] V. KOCHUPILLAI,[1] S. MATHEW,[1] N.K. MEHRA,[2] A. NANU,[3]
N. JAYASURYAN,[4] S. SHARMA,[1] S, FRANCIS[1] and P.S.N. MENON[1]

Medical Oncology Department, Institute Rotary Cancer Hospital, [1] Cytogenetic
Laboratory, Paediatrics Department, [2] HLA Laboratory, Anatomy Department, [3] Blood
Bank, [4] Radio-immuno assay Laboratory, Endocrinology Department, All India Institute
of Medical Sciences, New Delhi, IND-110029, India

Key words: fetal liver infusion, temporary engraftment, temporary mixed chimerism

Summary. Studies to find engraftment following fetal liver infusion (FLI) in aplastic anaemia
(AA) and acute myeloid leukaemia (AML) were carried out in 24 patients (17 AA and 7 AML
patients) out of the 56 who received FLI. HLA studies done in 13 patients (3 AA and
5 AML), repeatedly after FLI, showed no significant change in HLA antigen pattern before
and after FLI. Red cell antigen studies were done in five (1 AA and 4 AML) patients, 3 weeks
to 7 months after FLI. One patient with AML who was Rh negative prior to reinduction
chemotherapy became Rh positive two months after FLI; six months later he was Rh
negative again. In the remaining patients there was no change in red cell antigen pattern after
FLI. Radio-immuno-assay to detect alpha-fetoprotein levels, carried out in 10 (8 AA and
2 AML) patients repeatedly after FLI, demonstrated no increase. In 13 patients (8 AA and
5 AML) in whom there was a sex difference between donor and recipient, bone marrow
cultures for sex chromosomes revealed mixture of XX and XY cells in 3 male patients with
aplastic anaemia. One male patient with AML demonstrated complete engraftment after
induction chemotherapy and FLI: all the mitoses studied were of XX pattern. Engraftment
was however temporary as repeated studies revealed reversion to XY pattern. The present
work suggests that infusion of fetal liver cells may sometimes induce temporary chimerism
or engraftment in an adult host; in the majority of cases, however, engraftment could not be
established.

Introduction

Fetal liver infustion (FLI) has been attempted in aplastic anaemia [5, 7, 9],
acute leukaemia [8, 9] and severe combined immune deficiencies [1, 2, 6].
Although responses have been reported, the mechanism of bone marrow
recovery after FLI is not clear. We describe studies directed at detecting
evidence of engraftment of the fetal liver cells in responding individuals.

Materials and methods

Twenty-four patients, 17 with severe aplastic anaemia (AA) and 7 with
acute myeloid leukaemia (AML), who responded to fetal liver infusion
were studied. Details are presented elsewhere [9, 10]. Studies included

Address for offprints: Dr. Vinod Kochupillai, Associate Professor, Institute Rotary Cancer
Hospital, All India Institute of Medical Sciences, New Delhi, IND-110029, India.

HLA A, B and C typing, analysis of red cell antigens, alpha-fetoprotein levels and karyotype analysis.

HLA typing

HLA A, B and C antigens were tested according to the method of Terasaki and McCleland [15], in thirteen patients before and after fetal liver infusion. This included eight patients with AA and five with AML. Initial studies were done in 5–10 days after FLI and subsequently at an interval of 1–4 months.

Red cell antigens

Red cell antigens (ABO, Rh, MNS, Duffy and $Le^a Le^b$) were studied in five patients including one with AA and four with AML before and 3–4 weeks after FLI. Patients with AML often required large numbers of blood transfusions [8, 9] in addition to the infusion of fetal liver cells. Complete RBC typing of transfused units was not always available.

Alpha-fetoproteins (AFP)

Radio-immuno-assay (Lot No. 110, activity 4 mci, Amersham International) was utilized to determine levels of alpha-fetoprotein in 10 patients including 8 AA and 2 AML, before and after fetal liver infusion. Patient serum was collected every third day for ten days and then monthly for 2 to 8 months, and stored at − 20 °C. Samples were assayed on the same day in duplicate and reported in ng/ml.

Chromosome studies

Cytogenetic analysis was performed in 13 patients including 8 AA and 5 AML when there was a sex difference between donor and recipient

Table 1. Chromosomal analysis in aplastic anaemia after fetal liver infusion (FLI).

Case No.	Age (yrs)/ sex of patient	Age (weeks)/ sex of abortus	Chromosome analysis	Post-FLI days
1	12 M	10 F	54% (46 XX) 46% (46 XY)	5
3	43 M	16 F	(i) 60% (46 XX) 40% (46 XY)	114
			(ii) 100% (46 XY)	239
8	28 M	11 F	50% (46 XX) 50% (46 XY)	15
31	35 F	12.5 M	100% (46 XX)	180
33	10 M	13 F	100% (46 XY)	150
34	23 M	9 F	100% (46 XY)	30
37	27 M	17 F	100% (46 XY)	11
38	24 M	18 F	100% (46 XY)	45

Table 2. Chromosomal analysis in acute myeloid leukaemia after fetal liver infusion (FLI).

Case No.	Age (yrs)/ sex of patient	Age (weeks)/ sex of abortus	Chromosome analysis	Post-FLI days
1	32 M	20 F	(i) 100% (46 XX)	12
			(ii) 100% (46 XY)	30
3	23 M	19 F	100% (46 XY)	22
4	32 M	23 F	100% (46 XY)	60
13	45 F	18 M	100% (46 XX)	13
15	22 M	14 F	100% (46 XY)	85

(Tables 1 and 2). 0.5 ml of bone marrow aspirate was obtained in heparinized medium and incubated at 37 °C for 24 to 48 hours. Well spread metaphase preparations were made by standard techniques [14]. Briefly, it involved termination of bone marrow culture after 2 hours of colchicine (0.04 μg/ml) treatment at 37 °C. Cultures were harvested using 0.075 KCl. Methanol:acetic acid (3:1) fixative was added and slides, prepared by pouring 3 to 4 drops of the cell suspension onto a clean, 4 °C cold slide, were stained with 5% Giemsa. From each slide 15 to 30 well spread metaphases were analysed.

Results

HLA studies

None of the thirteen patients including 8 AA and 5 AML patients where HLA studies were carried out at repeated intervals, demonstrated change in HLA antigens after FLI [12].

Red cell antigens

Red cell antigen studies in five patients demonstrated no consistent change. One patient with AML who was Rh negative prior to fetal liver infusion became Rh positive two months later. When he was studied again in the 8th month, his red cells were Rh negative; this patient received extensive transfusion including Rh positive blood.

Alpha-fetoprotein

No demonstrable increase in the level of alpha-fetoprotein was detected in ten patients following fetal liver infusion.

Chromosome studies

Chromosome studies were performed in 13 patients in whom there was a sex difference between donor and recipient. Three male patients with AA showed mixture of XX and XY cells indicating chimerism after 5 to 114 days of the FLI (Table 1). In case 1, five days after the second fetal liver infusion, bone marrow cultures revealed cells with both XX (46) and XY (46) chromosomes, their percentages being 54 and 46 respectively. The marrow culture was analysed on the 114th day after the first FLI in case 3. It revealed both XX (46) and XY (46) types of chromosomes, their percentages being 60 and 40 respectively. The repeated study of patient 3 on the 239th post-FLI day showed that the chromosomal pattern had returned to XY in all 30 cells analysed. Marrow cultures analysed in case 8 on the 15th day after the second FLI revealed both XX (46) and XY (46) types of chromosomes, their percentage being 50% each. One male patient (case 1) with AML demonstrated complete engraftment after fetal liver infusion (Table 2); all the metaphases studied at day twelve were 46 XX. Four weeks later the karyotype of bone marrow cells was again 46 XY.

Discussion

Improvement in haematopoiesis has been reported following FLI in severe AA and AML [5, 7, 8, 9, 10, 11, 17]. It is not clear at present whether this improvement is related to engraftment of fetal liver derived haematopoietic stem cells or to a simulatory effect of the fetal liver cell infusion on residual haematopoietic stem cells of the recipient. Our study was designed to assess possible engraftment of fetal liver cells in the absence of intensive pre-transplant conditioning.

A common method of detecting engraftment is to study cytogenetics of bone marrow cells in transplants where the sexes of donor and recipient differ. Mixture of XX and XY cells in three of eight patients with AA indicates that fetal liver cells may temporarily engraft in some recipients. In one patient, however, mixture of XX and XY cells was observed on the 5th day after FLI. It is difficult to say whether this finding reflects true engraftment or persistence of donor fetal liver cells in the recipient's bone marrow. Temporary engraftment is clear in case 3 where mixture of XX and XY cells was observed on the 114th day after FLI. It is possible that temporary engraftment has also occurred in other patients but has not been detectable.

In one case of AML where fetal liver cells were infused after chemotherapy [8, 9], complete engraftment occurred. Engraftment was, however, temporary and the karyotype returned to host type within four weeks. In animal experiments [3, 4, 13] where pre-conditioning regimen is utilized, fetal liver cells can engraft completely in adult recipients. Rejection in such a situation, however, is not uncommon, possibly due to the lack of T cells in the fetal liver [3]. Similarly transplants of T-cell depleted bone marrow have a relatively high incidence of rejection.

In the majority of the patients that we studied, bone marrow recovery occurred without apparent engraftment of fetal liver cells [5, 7, 8, 9, 10]. Recovery in these individuals is most likely due to an effect on the patients' haematopoietic stem cells. This hypothesis is supported by the lack of change in HLA and red cell antigens in peripheral blood, suggesting that circulating blood cells after fetal liver infusion are recipient derived. The change from Rh negative to positive in one patient with AML may indicate temporary engraftment; however, this patient had received several units of Rh positive blood.

Levels of alpha-fetoprotein have been reported to be transiently elevated in patients with metabolic disorders and immune deficiency diseases as a result of fetal liver engraftment [16]. In the present study, however, no patient receiving fetal liver infusion demonstrated any significant increase in alpha-fetoprotein. Rise in the level of alpha-fetoprotein may be related to the number of hepatocytes infused; in the present study, fetal liver cell suspensions contained very few hepatocytes.

Our study suggests that temporary engraftment of fetal liver cells in an adult host is possible even in the absence of pre-conditioning. In most instances, however, bone marrow recovery appears related to stimulation of the patient's own haematopoietic stem cells by an as yet unknown mechanism. The possibility exists that fetal liver cells may be responsible for immunologic or hormonal modulation of the recipient's haematopoiesis.

Acknowledgements

The Department of Science and Technology financed this study. Dr. V. Kochupillai collaborated in the radioimmunoassay and Miss Vandana typed the manuscript. We acknowledge sincere thanks to Dr. R.P. Gale, Associate Professor of Medicine, University of California in Los Angeles, USA for his help in the preparation of this manuscript.

References

1. Bortin MM, Rimm AA (1977) Severe combined immunodeficiency disease. Characterization of the disease and results of tranplantation a, b, c. Seventh report from the International bone marrow transplant registry. J Am Med Ass 238:591–600
2. Buckley RH, Whisnant JK, Schiff RI, Gilbertsen RB, Huang AT, Platt MS (1976) Correction of severe combined immunodeficiency of fetal liver cells. New Engl J Med 294:1076–1081
3. Champlin R: Results of T-Lymphocyte depleted bone marrow transplantation. Implications for fetal liver transplants. Thymus (this issue)
4. Champlin R, Cain G, Stitizel K, Gale RP: Successful engraftment of MHC mismatched fetal liver hematopoietic cells in dogs. Thymus (this issue)
5. Kansal V, Sood SK, Batra AK, Adhar G, Malaviya AK, Kucheria K, Balakrishnan K (1979) Fetal liver transplantation in aplastic anaemia. Acta haematologica 62:128–136
6. Keightly RG, Lawton AR, Cooper MD (1975) Successful fetal liver transplantation in a child with severe combined immunodeficiency. Lancet 2:850–853
7. Kochupillai V, Sharma S, Francis S, Mehra NK, Nanu A, Kalra V, Menon PSN, Bhargava M (1985) Bone marrow reconstitution following human fetal liver infusion (FLI) in sixteen severe aplastic anaemia patients. In: Gale RP, Lucarelli G, Touraine JL, (eds) Fetal Liver Transplantation. New York: Alan R Liss, pp 251–265

8. Kochupillai V, Sharma S, Francis S, Mehra NK, Nanu A, Verma IC, Takkar D, Kumar S, Gokhale U (1985) Fetal liver infusion: An adjuvant in the therapy of acute myeloid leukaemia (AML). In: Gale RP, Touraine JL, Lucarelli G (eds) Fetal Liver Transplantation. New York: Alan R Liss, pp 267–279

9. Kochupillai V, Sharma S, Francis S, Nanu A, Verma IC, Bhatia P, Dua H, Kumar L, Aggarwal S, Singh S: Fetal liver infusion in acute myeloid leukaemia. Thymus (this issue)

10. Kochupillai V, Sharma S, Francis S, Nanu A, Mathew S, Bhatia P, Dua H, Kumar L, Aggarwal S, Singh S: Fetal liver infusion in aplastic anaemia. Thymus (this issue)

11. Lucarelli G, Izzi T, Porcellini A, Delfini C, Polchi P, Moretti L, Manna A, Grilli G (1980) Fetal Liver transplantation in aplastic anaemia and acute leukaemia. In: Lucarelli G, Fliedner TM, Gale RP (eds) Fetal Liver Transplantation. Current Concepts and future Directions, pp 284–299

12. Mehra NK, Taneja V, Jhingan B, Sharma S, Kochupillai V: HLA status following fetal liver transplantation in aplastic anaemia and acute myeloid leukaemia. Thymus (this issue)

13. Prummer O, Raghabachar A, Werner C, Clavo W, Carbonell F, Steinback I, Fliedner TM (1985) Fetal Liver Transplantation in Dogs. Transplantation 39:349–355

14. Srivastava AK, Smith RD (1980) A simple reliable procedure for obtaining metaphases from leukaemic bone marrow aspirates suitable for Giemsa banding. In Vitro 16:190–212

15. Terasaki PJ, McCleland JD (1964) Microdroplet assay of human serum cytotoxins. Nature 204:998–1000

16. Touraine JL (1980) Value of alpha-fetoprotein determination in the monitoring of patients with a fetal liver transplant for Fabry's disease or immunodeficiency. In: Lucarelli G, Fliedner TM, Gale RP (eds) Fetal Liver Transplantation. Current Concepts and future Directions. Amsterdam: Excerpta Medica, pp 300–302

17. Wu CT, Ye GY: Advances in experimental studies and clinical applications of fetal liver cells. Thymus (this issue)

Thymus 10:131–136 (1987)
© Martinus Nijhoff Publishers, Dordrecht

HLA status following fetal liver transplantation in aplastic anaemia and acute myeloid leukaemia

N.K. MEHRA,[1] V. TANEJA,[1] B. JHINGHON,[1] T. CHAUDHURI,[1] S. SHARMA[2] and V. KOCHUPILLAI[2]

[1] Cellular Immunology Laboratory, Department of Anatomy; and [2] Medical Oncology Department, All India Institute of Medical Sciences, New Delhi, IND — 110 029, India

Summary. Fetal liver infusion (FLI) was tried as an alternate mode of therapy in 40 patients with aplastic anaemia and in 16 patients with acute myeloid leukaemia. The fetal HLA typing carried out on spleen and thymus cells revealed that, while it was more difficult to HLA type the thymus than the spleen cells, 'full house' antigens could be determined only in fetuses of 18 weeks or older. No special effort was made to transfuse HLA- matched or partially matched donor cells into the recipient. The recipients were HLA typed at varying time intervals following FLI in an attempt to document a possible chimerism. None of the patients revealed a 'shift' in their HLA antigen profile and there was no evidence of any donor cell engraftment. No relationship between the HLA match of donor and recipient, and the general condition, the prognosis or the total survival of the patient was evidenced. These data indicate that, even though fetal liver cells express HLA antigens, these cells are functionally incompetent to cause an apparent graft-versus-host disease in the host.

Introduction

Though bone marrow transplantation is an effective treatment for a number of immunologic and haematologic disorders including severe aplastic anaemia [1] and possibly acute myeloid leukaemia, it suffers from the serious disadvantage of its cost and from the poor results when no HLA- matched family donor is available. Also, graft-versus-host disease (GvHD) and infections are severe complications in patients with successful marrow engraftment. Fetal liver has been employed as an alternative source of haematopoietic stem cells both in experimental animals [1] as well as in humans [4,5]. The liver is the major site of haematopoiesis during the second trimester of gestation and it is virtually devoid of mature T-lymphocytes.

In the present study, fetal liver infusion (FLI) has been tried as an alternative mode of therapy in patients with aplastic anaemia (AA) and acute myeloid leukaemia (AML). The HLA status of the donor grafted cells as well as of the recipient's before and after FLI was determined. The study was conducted with the following aims: (i) to assess 'engraftment' of donor cells by the host; (ii) to understand the possible influence of HLA

Address for offprints: Dr. N.K. Mehra, Assistant Professor, Cellular Immunology Laboratory, Department of Anatomy, All India Institute of Medical Sciences, New Delhi, IND — 110 029, India.

compatibility between the donor and the recipient on the success of the fetal liver transplant; and (iii) to observe the beneficial effects of FLI in the recipients.

Materials and methods

During the period between late 1976 and November 1985, a total of 56 patients received FLI. Forty of these patients were diagnosed to have AA and 16 AML. The diagnosis of AA was made by the peripheral blood findings, bone marrow aspiration and bone marrow biopsy which was markedly hypocellular in all of them.

The diagnosis of AML was made on the peripheral blood picture and confirmed on bone marrow examination.

Fetuses were obtained from patients in whom abortion was induced by intra-amniotic prostaglandin administration, or hysterotomy. Fetuses ranged in age between 12 weeks and 22 weeks. Fetal liver cells for infusion were prepared according to the method already described [4].

HLA typing

HLA typing of the fetal donor was carried out on lymphocytes obtained from the spleen and from the thymus, removed under sterile conditions. A single cell suspension was made by syringing into RPMI-1640 culture medium. Viability of the cells was checked by the trypan blue exclusion method. The lymphocytes thus obtained were adjusted to a concentration of 2×10^6 cells per ml and typed for HLA class I antigens (A, B & C loci) using the standard two stage NIH microlymphocytotoxicity technique [8]. For typing of fetal cells, the incubation period was increased from 30 minutes to 45 minutes for the first stage (cells + antiserum) and from 60 minutes to 90 minutes for the 2nd stage (after addition of complement).

Out of the fifty-six patients, 30 patients (22 AA and 8 AML) were HLA typed, following FLI, at varying time intervals up to three years. The first post-FLI HLA typing was done within one to three weeks of infusion and repeated at intervals of 1–4 months.

Results

HLA typing of the fetal thymus cells presented more difficulties than that of the fetal spleen cells. It is known that only the medullary thymocytes express HLA antigens [3] and that class I MHC antigens are expressed at reduced levels on the majority of thymocytes (6). In the younger fetuses, e.g. 12–16 weeks, only 25–50% HLA antigens could be detected while

Table 1. HLA typing in fetal spleen and thymus.

Gestational age	Spleen	Thymus
12 wks*	A3?	–
14 wks*	A1	A1
16 wks*	A9, B12	
18 wks		A28, A30, B35, B40
20 wks	A9, A11, B35	
21 wks	A1, A9, B35, B40, Cw2	
22 wks		A3, A11, B5, B62, Cw3

* Parental HLA typing done in these cells.

'full house' HLA phenotyping was possible in fetuses after 18 weeks of gestation (Table 1). In some fetuses, the HLA phenotypes were confirmed by parental HLA typing.

Eight of the 22 patients in the AA group and 5 of the 8 in the AML group were followed for their HLA antigen profile. Table 2 shows the pre- and post-transplant HLA status in AA patients following FLI. None of these patients revealed a shift in their HLA profile and there was no evidence of any chimerism with donor cells. In two patients, full HLA antigens corresponding to the pre-graft stage could not be detected immediately following fetal liver infusion. This was due to weak serological reactivity of the recipient cells. One patient (H.S.B.) showed temporary expression of Cw3 antigen (cells of fetal origin). This patient had also shown evidence of temporary chimerism on chromosomal studies [4]. Similar findings were observed for the AML group of patients who also showed lack of stable donor cell engraftment.

An attempt was made to correlate the general condition, the prognosis and the total survival of the patient with the grade of HLA matching between the donor and the recipient. The data for AA and AML are shown in Tables 3 and 4 respectively. In the former, one patient (HSB) who received 50% match grade fetal liver cells had the longest survival of 106 months. Two other patients (Vinod and ASK) received poorly

Table 2. Pre- and post-transplant HLA status in aplastic anaemia following liver infusion.

Patient total = 23	No. of FLI	HLA Antigens of Recipient			
		Pre-Graft	Post-Graft		
			I	II	Subsequent
BS	Three	9, 19, 7, Cw1	No change	–	–
ML	Three	9, 19, 33, 8	No change	–	–
Vinod	One	11, 35, 40, Cw3	No change	–	–
HSB	Three	9, 19, 35, 40, Cw4	Temp. engraftment of Cw3	–	–
ASK	One	9, 26, 5, 35	Less antigens	–	–
MB	Two	1, 19, 17, 40, Cw3	No change	–	–
KKG	One	3, 28, 18, 27	No change	–	–
JLP	One	9, 7, 40	Less antigens	–	–

Table 3. Relationship between HLA compatibility and prognosis following FLI in aplastic anaemia.

Fetal liver HLA	Name	HLA	Compatibility %	Marrow cellularity	G.C.	Fever	Blood transfusion	Survival (months)
9, 11, 5, 44	Vinod	11, 35, 40, Cw3	25	Normal	Good	−	Nil	36 M (alive)
1, 9, 17, 40	HSB	9, 19, 35, 40, Cw4	50	Normal	Good	±	Occasional	106 M (dead)
2, 40	ASK	9, 26, 5, 35	Nil	Normal	Good	−	Nil	42 M (alive)
1, 2, 17, 40	JLP	9, 19, 7, 40	25	No response	Poor	+	Plenty	2 M (dead)
2, 5, 22, Cw2	KKG	3, 28, 18, 27	Nil	Partial response	Moder.	+	Plenty	5 M (dead)

G.C. = general condition some weeks after FLI

Table 4. Relationship between HLA compatibility and prognosis following FLI in acute myeloid leukaemia.

Fetal liver HLA	Patient Name	HLA	Compatibility %	Prognosis Remission	G.C	Fever	Blood Transf.	Survival (months)
1, 9, 35, 40, Cw2	KC	11, 32, 35, Cw4	25	Complete	Good	−	Nil*	32 M (dead)
28, 30, 35, 40	VS	1, 11, 35, 37, Cw4	25	Complete	Good	−	Nil*	20 M (dead)
3, 11, 5, 62, Cw3	SS	1, 9, 37, 62, Cw4	25	Complete	Good	−	Nil*	28 M (dead)
	GD	9, 33, 5, 7	−	Partial	Moder.	−	Nil*	3 M (dead)
9, 11, 35, Cw4	MPG	19, 17, 35, Cw4	50	Nil	Poor	+	Plenty	2 M (dead)

* Blood transfusions given during induction only.
G.C. = general condition some weeks after FLI.

matched cells, but showed good prognosis and are still alive. None of these three patients was transfusion dependent. Indeed, the two patients (HLP and KKG) who required plenty of blood transfusions following FLI had very poor prognosis.

In the AML group of patients also, no relationship between HLA compatibility of the donor-recipient pair and overall prognosis was observed.

Discussion

Though HLA antigens are known to be expressed on the nucleated cells very early during intra-uterine life, it is not possible to detect the full phenotype (including HLA-DR) until 18 weeks of gestation, using the conventional NIH microlymphocytotoxicity technique [2]. In the present study, no attempt at matching the fetal donors and the patients was made, so that only one or two antigens in the HLA-A, B, and C loci were shared between donor cells and host. No evidence of a permanent chimerism with mixed HLA types was visible in any of the recipients despite more than one FLI in some cases. It is pertinent to note that these patients were given FLI without any pre-conditioning with large doses of chemotherapy and total body irradiation. These data indicate that the infusion of fetal liver cells provides a temporary stimulus to the patient's own bone marrow for regeneration. This effect was clearly visible in the AA group of patients. In some cases, where regeneration didn't occur, repeated FLIs were necessary to ensure prolonged survival. The mechanism by which the infused fetal liver cells bring about regeneration of the host's own haematopoietic tissue is not clear though possibility for the existence of an 'haemopoiesis modulating factor' in the fetal liver cannot be ruled out. In this context, beneficial effects following successive injections of fetal liver extract in the AA group has been reported [4].

The absence of GvHD despite infusion with HLA mismatched cells in the AA and in the AML groups indicates that, even though fetal liver cells express HLA antigens, they are functionally incompetent in inducing this severe reaction, presumably because the fetal liver is virtually devoid of mature T-lymphocytes.

Acknowledgements

The financial assistance for the project was given by the Indian Council of Medical Research (ICMR) and the Department of Science and Technology (DST), Government of India. The authors wish to thank the Department of Obstetrics and Gynaecology for their help in procuring fetuses.

References

1. Bortin MM, Rimm AA, Rose WC, Tritt RL, Saltzstein EC (1976) Transplantation of haematopoietic and lymphoid cells in mice. Transplantation 21:331–336
2. Danilovs JA, Brown J, Terasaki PI, Clark WR (1983) HLA-DR and HLA-A, B and C typing of human fetal tissue. Tissue antigens 21:296–308
3. Janossy G, Thomas JA, Bollum FJ, Granger S, Pizzolo G, Bradstock KF, Wong L, McMichael A, Ganeshaguru K, Hoffbrand AV (1980) The human thymic microenvironment: An immunohistologic study. J Immunol 125:202–212
4. Kansal V, Sood SK, Batra AK, Adhar G, Malaviya AN, Kucheria K, Balakrishnan K (1979) Fetal liver transplantation in aplastic anaemia. Acta Haematologica 62:128–136
5. Lucarelli G, Izzi T, Porcellini A et al. (1980) Fetal liver transplantation in aplastic anaemia and acute leukaemia. In: G Lucarelli, TM Fliedner, RP Gale (eds) Fetal Liver Transplantation. Current Concepts and Future Directions. Excerpta Medica, p 285
6. Scollay R, Jacobs S, Jerabek L, Butcher E, Weissman I T cell maturation: [(1980)] Thymocyte and thymus migrant subpopulations defined with monoclonal antibodies to MHC region antigens. J Immunol 124:2845–2853
7. Storb R. Prentice RL, Buckner CD, Clift RA, Appelbaum F, Deeg J, Doney K, Hansen JA, Mason M, Sanders JE, Singer J, Sullivan KM, Witherspoon RP, Thomas ED (1983) Graft-versus-host disease and survival in patients with aplastic anaemia treated by marrow grafts fro HLA-identical siblings. New Eng J Med 308:302–307
8. Terasaki PI, McCleland JD (1964) Microdroplet assay of human serum cytotoxins. Nature (Lond) 204:998–1000
9. Wu-Chu-tse et al.: Studies on the mechanism of fetal liver transfusion or whole fetal liver extract injection in the treatment of anaemia. Thymus (this issue).

Thymus 10:137–146 (1987)
© Martinus Nijhoff Publishers, Dordrecht

Marrow uptake index (MUI): A quantitative scintigraphic study of bone marrow in aplastic anaemia

A.K. PADHY, A. GARG,[1] V. KOCHUPILLAI,[2] P.G. GOPINATH and A.K. BASU

All India Institute of Medical Sciences New Delhi, IND-110029, India; Dept. of Nuclear Medicine; [1] Dept. of Medicine; [2] Dept. of Medical Oncology (I.R.C.H)

Key words: aplastic anaemia, dynamic bone marrow imaging, bone marrow uptake index

Summary. Aplastic anaemia affects the entire bone marrow. Current methods of assessment of bone marrow function, like bone marrow biopsy or peripheral blood examination are either invasive or inadequate and cannot be expected to represent fully the changes in the entire bone marrow tissue. This prospective study was undertaken to develop and standardise a new Nuclear Medicine technique called 'Dynamic Bone marrow Imaging'.

Eleven patients and ten controls were studied. Serial images of the pelvis were obtained in frame mode following intravenous injection of 185–370 mBq of ^{99m}Tc S. Colloid, and an index, called the Bone Marrow Uptake Index (P) was calculated by taking into consideration the time activity curve obtained over the iliac crest. This was followed by static imaging of the entire bone marrow in all cases.

It was possible to obtain excellent information regarding topographic distribution of bone marrow as well as detect early changes in bone marrow function following treatment. An attempt was also made to correlate bone marrow cellularity as obtained by bone marrow biopsy with the results of dynamic bone marrow scintigraphy. On the basis of the encouraging results obtained in the present study, the authors feel that dynamic bone marrow imaging is an excellent technique for the objective evaluation of bone marrow in aplastic anaemia.

Aplastic anaemia affects the entire bone marrow tissue. Although much progress has been made in the management of this disease, many aspects of it await better understanding. There is almost total lack of knowledge regarding the distribution of functioning marrow in various phases of aplastic anaemia, such as in relapse and remission [1, 2, 6, 10, 20]. Current methods of assessment of marrow function rely mainly on bone marrow biopsy and peripheral blood examination. Bone marrow biopsy is invasive and cannot be expected to represent fully the changes in the entire tissue [4]. Changes in peripheral blood picture lag behind the changes in the bone marrow. Thus, there is a need for an investigation which is safe, simple, sensitive, non invasive and capable of assessing the global function of bone marrow.

Radio-nuclide imaging of bone marrow requires labelling of one or more components of this widely dispersed tissue. The reticuloendothelial and erythropoietic components can be labelled with radio-colloids and radio-iron respectively [3, 5, 8, 9, 12, 13, 15, 16, 17, 19]. Experimental studies have shown that the reticuloendothelial and erythropoietic elements are invariably found together in the marrow and have similar distribution [7, 18].

This report is based on a prospective study of bone marrow function in patients with aplastic anaemia, using ^{99m}Tc. Sulphur colloid.

Materials and methods

Eleven patients (8 males and 3 females) with aplastic anaemia were included in the study. All patients selected for this study fulfilled the follow-

Address for offprints: Dr. A.K. Padhy, Dept. of Nuclear Medicine, A.I.I.M.S., IND-110029 New Delhi, India.

ing diagnostic criteria: (1) Polymorphnuclear cell count less than 500/ mm^3; (2) Reticulocyte count less than 1%, (3) Duration of symptoms less than six months; and (4) Markedly hypocellular marrow on bone marrow biopsy [11]. Ages ranged between 14 and 40 years with a mean age of 27.4 years. On the same day, prior to bone marrow scintigraphy, these patients were evaluated in the following manner: (1) Thorough clinical examination; (2) Peripheral blood examination including an estimation of hemoglobin, reticulocyte count, total leucocyte, neutrophil and platelet counts; (3) Bone marrow biopsy to study marrow cellularity.

The control group in this study consisted of ten patients (8 males and 2 females) who attended the Nuclear Medicine Department for liver scintigraphy. Their ages ranged between 15 and 42 years with a mean age of 26.8 years. Significant haematological disorders in these patients were ruled out by thorough physical examination and routine haematological tests which included estimation of hemoglobin level, total and differential leucocyte counts, total platelet count and peripheral smear for cell morphology.

A total of 35 bone marrow scintigraphy studies were done in both the control and aplastic anaemia patients (Table 1). In 5 patients with anaemia it was possible to do bone marrow imaging before and after treatment. In the rest, it was possible to conduct only post-treatment imaging. The treatment consisted of androgens and fetal liver cell infusion (FLI) as described by Kochupillai et al. [11]. Some patients had more than one study following treatment. The results of bone marrow scintigraphy were correlated with clinical and haematological features including bone marrow biopsy.

The technique of dynamic bone marrow imaging is as follows: The patient is placed prone under the gamma camera with pelvis facing the centre of the detector. A dose of about 185–370 mBq ^{99m}Tc. Sulphur Colloid is injected intravenously as a bolus and scintigraphic data are collected using the standard soft-ware of a computer in frame mode (120 frames, time per frame being 8 seconds). Regions of interest are selected over the iliac bone and over the background of the soft tissues. Area normalised, background substracted, time activity curves are generated

Table 1. Bone marrow scintigraphy in aplastic anaemia.

		No. of studies
1.	Control group	10
2.	Aplastic anaemia group	
	Before treatment	6
	After treatment (before full recovery)	15
	After full recovery	4

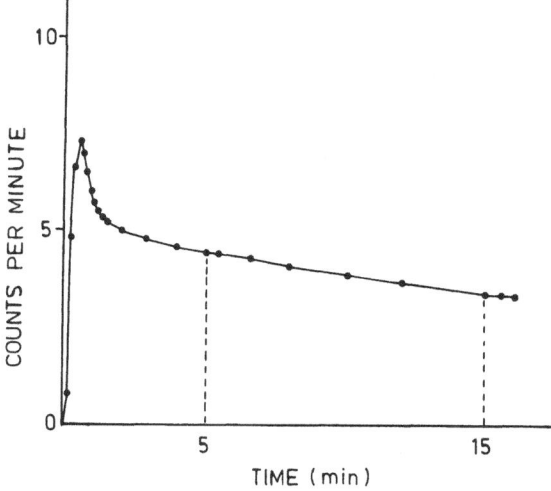

Figure 1. ⁹⁹ᵐTc. S. Colloid dynamic bone marrow scintigraphy. Background substracted time activity curve over the right iliac crest obtained in a control subject. Marrow uptake index is determined by calculating the ratio of the counts at 15 minutes over counts at 5 minutes.

over selected regions of interest (Figure 1). Taking into consideration the time activity curve obtained over the iliac bone, a ratio of counts at 15 minutes over the counts at 5 minutes is calculated. This value is called the bone marrow uptake index (P). Immediately following the acquisition of the time activity curve, static bone marrow images of the body are obtained, which include those in the skull, near the shoulder joints, chest wall, axial skeleton, pelvis and near the hip joints (Figure 2).

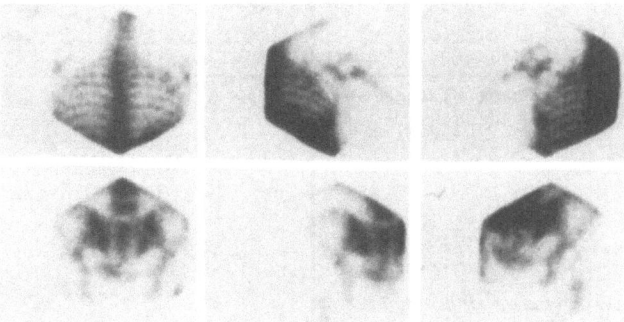

Figure 2. ⁹⁹ᵐTc. S. Colloid bone marrow scintigraphy in a control subject. Static images. All posterior views. Clock-wise from top left: images of thorax, right shoulder, left shoulder, pelvis, left hip joint and right hip joint. Scans show good uptake, uniform distribution and normal extent of bone marrow activity.

140

Results

The results of the bone marrow scintigraphy were categorised according to the classification given in Table 2. This is a modified version of the classification suggested by McNeal et al. [14]. All ten control subjects showed good uptake of radio-colloid by the bone marrow with uniform distribution, allowing sharp delineation of bone marrow tissue. In all these cases the marrow activity was found to be confined to proximal humerus, proximal femur, pelvis, vertebrae, ribs, scapulae, sternum and the skull (Figure 2). The range of bone marrow uptake index in controls was found to be between 0.76 and 0.87 (mean $\pm$ S.D. $= 0.80 \pm 0.05$).

Results obtained in patients were analysed taking into consideration three parameters: (1) Radio-colloid uptake by the bone marrow: (2) Extent of distribution; and (3) Bone marrow uptake index (Table 2).

Radio-colloid uptake by bone marrow

A spectrum of bone marrow uptake patterns was observed in this series. These were classified into five distinct categories. They are as follows:
   (a) Absent Uptake: No radio-colloid uptake in the bone marrow.
   (b) Minimal Uptake: Radio-colloid uptake just above body background.
   (c) Bone marrow well delineated: Radio-colloid uptake in marrow better than 'b', but less than normal.
   (d) Normal uptake: Radio-colloid uptake in the marrow allowing sharp delineation of the organ comparable with the quality of images obtained in normal control subjects.
   (e) More than normal uptake: Characterised by islands with focally increased uptake of radio-colloid.

Table 2. Classification of bone marrow scan.

I.	*Radio-coloid uptake* Less than normal	
		— a (Absent uptake)
		— b (Mineral uptake)
		— c (Bone marrow well delineated)
	Normal	— d
	More than normal	— e
II.	*Extent of distribution* Normal	— a
	Expanded	— b
	Contracted	— c
III.	Bone marrow uptake index (P).	

Extent of radio-colloid distribution

The extent of distribution of radio-colloid in the bone marrow of patients with aplastic anaemia as seen on static imaging was classified as follows:
  (a) Normal: Presence of radio-colloid uptake at normal anatomic sites as determined by studies in controls.
  (b) Expanded: Presence of bone marrow activity at additional sites, where radio-colloid uptake by bone marrow is normally absent.
  (c) Contracted: Absent bone marrow activity from proximal ends of femur and humerus.

Bone marrow uptake index (P)

Bone marrow uptake index (P) was calculated using the formula given below:

$$P = \frac{\text{Counts obtained over iliac bone at 15 minutes}}{\text{Counts obtained over iliac bone at 05 minutes}}$$

In control subjects the range of 'P' was between 0.76 and 0.87 (Mean: 0.80). In all cases of aplastic anaemia the bone marrow uptake index was found to be less than the normal value.

In six patients with aplastic anaemia, bone marrow scintigraphy was done prior to institution of therapy. These six patients had moderately severe peripheral pancytopenia and markedly hypocellular marrow on biopsy. All of them revealed contracted marrow with invariable absence of radio-colloid concentration in the proximal ends of femora and humeri. They also revealed generalised reduced radio-colloid uptake with a simultaneously low marrow uptake index, values ranging between 0.55 and 0.71 (Figure 3). Table 3 shows the results of bone marrow biopsy and bone marrow scintigraphy in these patients.

Results of haematological examination, bone marrow biopsy and bone marrow scintigraphy in four patients who were studied both before and after treatment with FLI but before the onset of complete haematological recovery is given in Table 4. It was observed that following institution of therapy there was no improvement in peripheral blood parameters in any patient. In one of these patients bone marrow biopsy showed hypercellularity. Bone marrow scintigraphy also revealed expanded marrow with multiple islands of hyperactive marrow in both femora with high bone marrow uptake index. This patient subsequently recovered fully after six months. In three other patients bone marrow remained hypocellular but bone marrow imaging revealed good uptake and normal marrow uptake index.

Four patients were studied after full recovery following FLI. All these patients revealed a normal peripheral blood study, normocellular marrow and normal features in radio-nuclide bone marrow scintigraphy (Figure 4) including a normal bone marrow uptake index (Table 5).

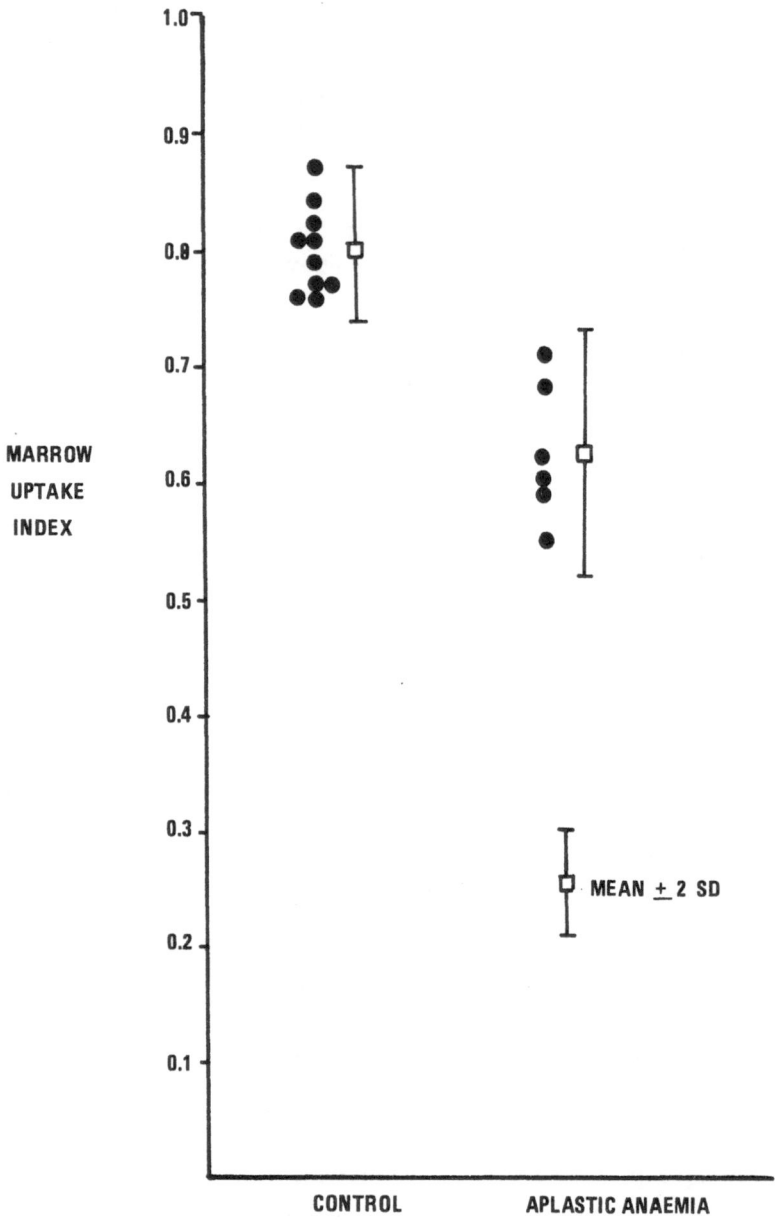

Figure 3. Bone marrow uptake index in control subjects (N:10) and in patients with aplastic anaemia (N:6) at diagnosis. Patients with aplastic anaemia have significantly lower marrow uptake index as compared to the control subjects (p < 0.001).

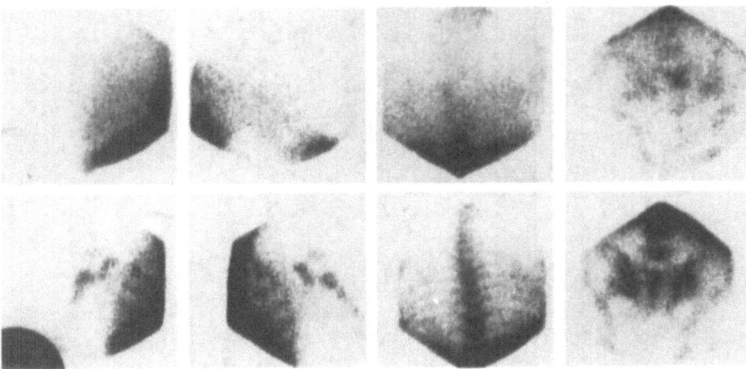

Figure 4. ^{99m}Tc. S. Colloid bone marrow scans in a patient with severe aplastic anaemia. Top row: Pre-treatment scans. From left to right: left shoulder, right shoulder, thorax and pelvis. These scans show very poor uptake of radio-colloid, gross patchy distribution and absence of marrow activity in the proximal ends of humeri on both sides. Bottom row: Scans in the same patient six months after FLI. Scans, arranged in the same order as in the top row, demonstrate uptake patterns comparable with those of normal controls.

Discussion

One of the important observations in the present study is the alteration in the topographic distribution of functioning marrow in cases of aplastic anaemia. All six patients studied before the institution of any treatment showed contracted marrow invariably in the form of total absence of activity in the proximal ends of long bones (femora, humeri). The marrow uptake index was also found to be significantly low as compared to the results obtained in the control group (Figure 3). These findings correlated well with the observations made in the peripheral blood examination and bone marrow biopsy done on the same day (Table 3).

All four patients studied after full haematological recovery showed normal patterns both in the uptake and extent of activity. Similar observations have also been reported by other investigators using ^{111}In. chloride [16, 18].

Table 3. Bone marrow cellularity and results of bone marrow scintigraphy in patients with aplastic anaemia at diagnosis

Serial no.	Results of bone marrow biopsy	Results of bone marrow scintigraphy		
		Uptake	Extent	Bone marrow uptake index
1.	Markedly hypocellular marrow	Less than normal	contracted	0.55
2.	-do-	Less than normal	contracted	0.71
3.	-do-	Less than normal	contracted	0.68
4.	-do-	Less than normal	contracted	0.68
5.	-do-	Less than normal	contracted	0.60
6.	-do-	Less than normal	contracted	0.59

Table 4. Correlation between changes in haematological profile, bone marrow cellularity and results of bone marrow scintigraphy in patients with aplastic anaemia before and after therapy, but prior to full recovery.

Serial no.	Peripheral blood picture		Bone marrow biopsy		Marrow scintigraphy						Clinical					
					Uptake		Extent		Uptake index		Blood transfusion units/month		Hemorrhage		infection	
	Pre	Post	Pre	Post	Pre	Post	Pre	Post	Pre	Post	Pre	Post	Pre	Post	Pre	Post
1.	No change	No change	No change		b	d	c	c	0.68	0.89	3	1	+	−	−	−
2.	No change	No change	No change		b	d	c	a	0.71	0.90	3	1	+	−	+	−
3.	No change	No change	No change		b	d	c	a	0.60	0.90	4	0	+	−	−	−
4.	No change	No change	No change		b	e	c	b	0.55	1.04	3	0	+	−	+	−

Pre: Before therapy
Post: After therapy
+: Present
−: Absent

Table 5. Haematological profile, bone marrow cellularity and results of bone marrow scintigraphy after full recovery following treatment

Case no.	Blood	Bone marrow cellularity	Bone marrow scintigraphy		
			Uptake	Extent	Marrow uptake index
1	Normal	Normo cellular	Normal	Normal	0.79
2	Normal	Normo cellular	Normal	Normal	0.83
3	Normal	Normo cellular	Normal	Normal	0.81
4	Normal	Normo cellular	Normal	Normal	0.77

Four patients who were studied 3–4 months after fetal liver infusion (Table 4) continued to have severe pancytopenia and all but one continued to have markedly hypocellular marrow. In all these patients the blood transfusion requirements and the frequency of haemorrhagic and infectious complications were significantly reduced following FLI. At the same time the bone marrow scintigraphy revealed normal or more than normal bone marrow uptake index. All these four patients subsequently showed further clinical improvement and went on to complete recovery within six months to one year. Hence, it appears that the improvement in bone marrow topography and uptake index occurs much before any appreciable change in bone marrow cellularity and peripheral blood parameters. Therefore marrow imaging may be a more sensitive tool than the conventional methods like marrow biopsy or peripheral blood examination in detecting early changes in bone marrow function following treatment.

Thus, the analysis of results in this prospective study offers a new diagnostic approach which can be employed in the initial assessment and subsequent follow-up of cases of aplastic anaemia. This technique is non-invasive. It appears to be a more sensitive and objective method than the conventional bone marrow biopsy for the detection of early changes in bone marrow function. Besides, it has the added advantage of low radiation dose to the patient, and hence can be repeated at relatively frequent intervals of time for serial evaluation of bone marrow function.

Acknowledgements

We are extremely grateful to Dr. K. Gopal Reddy, Senior resident in the department of Nuclear Medicine for his constructive suggestions; to Mrs Krishna Gupta and Mr Jaipal Singh for their excellent technical support.

References

1. Boggs DR, Boggs SS: The pathogenesis of Aplastic anaemia Blood 48:71–76, 1976
2. Dacie JV, Lewis SM: Practical Haematology (4th Edition) Churchill, London, 1968
3. Edward LC, Andrews GA, Sitterson BW, et al.: Clinical bone marrow scanning with radio isotopes Blood 23:741–756

4. Firsch B, Lewis SM: The bone marrow in aplastic anaemia: Diagnostic and prognostic features J Clin Pathol 27:231–241, 1974

5. Fordham EW, Amjad Ali: Radio nuclide imaging of the bone marrow Semin Hematol 18:222–239, 1981

6. Gale RP, Champlin RE, Feig SA, et al.: Aplastic anaemia: Biology and treatment Ann Intern Med 95:477–494, 1981

7. Greenberg ML, Atkins HL, Schiffer LM: Erythropoietic and reticuloendothelial fucntion in bone marrow in dogs Science 152:526–528, 1966

8. Henry RE, Fletcher JW, George EA, et al.: Bone marrow Tc.99m Sulphur Colloid distribution and marrow cellularity Am J Med Sci 270:419–424, 1975

9. Knisely RM: Marrow studies with radio colloids Semin Nucl Med 2:71–85, 1972

10. Kochupillai V, Sharma S, Sundaram KR: Anabolic steroids in aplastic anaemia Indian J Med Res 80:174–179, 1984

11. Kochupillai V, Sharma S, Francis S, et al.: Bone marrow reconstitution following human fetal liver infusion (FLI) in sixteen severe aplastic anaemia patients In Fetal Liver Transplantation, Ed. Gale RP and Touraine JL Alan R Liss, Inc, New York, 1985, p 251–265

12. Lillien DL, Berger HG, Andorson DP, et al.: Indium-111 Chloride: A new agent for bone marrow imaging J Nucl Med 14:184–186, 1973

13. McNeil BJ, Rappaport JM, Nattan DG: Indium chloride scintigraphy and index of severity in patients with aplastic anaemia Br J Haematol 34:599–604, 1976

14. McNeil BJ, Holman BL, Button LN, et al.: Use of Indium Chloride scintigraphy in patients of myelofibrosis J Nucl Med 15:647–651, 1974

15. Najean Y, Le Danvic M, Le Mercier N, et al.: Significance of bone marrow scintigraphy in aplastic anaemia- Concise communication. J Nucl Med 21:213–218, 1980

16. Neal LH, Bennett LR, Marciano RT: Evaluation of aplastic anaemia with In-111 Chloride Arch Intern Med 140:1299–1303, 1980

17. Nelp WB, Larson SM, Lewis RJ: Disribution of the erythron and RES in the bone marrow organ J Nucl Med 8: 430–434, 1967

18. Sayle BA, Helmer RE, Birdsong BA, et al.: Bone marrow imaging with In-111 Chloride in aplastic anaemia and myelofibrosis — Concise communication J Nucl Med 23:121–125, 1982

19. Schreiner DP: Reticuloendothelial scan in disorders involving the bone marrow J Nucl Med 15:1158–1162, 1974

20. Vincent PC, deGruchy GC: Complications and treatment of acquired aplastic anaemia Br J Haematol 13:977–999, 1967

Thymus 10:147–158 (1987)
© Martinus Nijhoff Publishers, Dordrecht

A comparison between ALG and bone marrow transplantation in treatment of severe aplastic anemia

BRUNO SPECK, ALOIS GRATWOHL, CATHERINE NISSEN, BRUNO
OSTERWALDER, ANDREAS WÜRSCH, ANDRÉ TICHELLI, ALFRED LORI,
PIERRE REUSSER, MICHEL JEANNET** and ERICH SIGNER*

Division of Hematology, Department of Internal Medicine, Kantonsspital, University of
Basel/Switzerland; * Kinderspital, University of Basel/Switzerland and; ** Division of
Transplantation Immunology, Hôpital Cantonal, Geneva, Switzerland

Key words: aplastic anemia, antilymphocyte globulin, bone marrow transplantation

Summary. One hundred patients with severe aplastic anemia were treated and evaluated in a prospective study at our hospital between January 1976 and October 1983. 28 patients had a HLA-identical sibling donor and were treated with bone marrow transplantation. 72 patients without a HLA-indentical sibling donor were given antilymhocyte globulin followed by oral low dose androgen therapy. One and a half years to nine years after treatment 13 patients (46%) survive in the transplant group and 53 patients (74%) survive in the second group. All except one in the second group have self-sustaining hematopoiesis without need for transfusions. There is one major difference between the two therapies. Marrow transplantation restores bone marrow function completely and no late hematological complications hav been seen in this group. The majority of patients treated with antilymphocyte globulin in contrast have residual abnormalities of hemopoliesis: macrocytosis, mild granulocytopenia and mild thrombocytopenia. Relapse (11 of 72 patients) and clonal hematological disorders, such as paroxysmal nocturnal hemoglobinuria (4 patients) and leukemia (one patient) can occur years after complete bone marrow reconsitution with antilymphocyte globulin. These late disorders are of concern. In spite of this we conclude that antilymphyocyte globulin treatment is an effective therapy with low early mortality and morbidity and a high chance for a long sustained remission. Results are better or at least equivalent to bone marrow transplantation and patients with donors should be given the option of transplantation or antilymphocyte globulin.

Introduction

Acquired severe aplastic anemia were evaluated as pancytopenia due to bone marrow failure [1]. The pathogenesisis unknown, although insight has been obtained from the results of the various therapeutic approaches. Aplastic anemia can be cured by replacement of hemopoietic tissue with bone marrow transplantation as well as reconstitution of autologous bone marrow function by antilymphocyte globulin therapy [1, 30]. Thus, a defect intrinsic to the hemopoietic stem cell and immune mechanisms extrinsic to the stem cell appear to be involved in its pathophysiology. So far the choice of treatment for individual patients has been determined by the availability of a histocompatible donor and by the age of the recipient. No randomized prospective study compared bone marrow transplanta-

Address for offprints: Bruno Speck, Kantonsspital Basel, Petersgraben 4, CH-4031 Basel, Switzerland.

tion with antilymphocyte globulin therapy. In 1981 we published the results of a prospective study comparing bone marrow transplantation and treatment with antilymphocyte globulin depending on the availability of a donor [19]. We showed that antilymphocyte globulin therapy assures survival at least as effectively as bone marrow transplantation. Open questions remained at that time and we continued the study. Today we can evaluate 100 patients treated at our institute and define the advantage and limitations of both treatment modalities.

Patients and methods

Study design

A prospective study was initiated in 1976. Until October 1983 100 patients with severe aplastic anemia have entered the study and have been treated at our hospital. Details of classification criteria and treatment have been previously published [19]. Essentially, patients up to the age of 40 years with a histocompatible sibling donor, matched at the HLA–A, –B and –DR–locus were treated with bone marrow transplantation, all other patients were treated with antilymphocyte globulin. Treatment protocols and their changes during the study due to experience and availability of new drugs are shown on Table 1.

Patients

Most patients were referred from other medical centers after failure of conventional treatment with low or high dose steroids and anabolic hormones. The two groups of patients (treated with bone marrow transplantation = group A, treated with antilymphocyte globulin = group B) are otherwise comparable in terms of patient age, etiology of aplastic anemia and severity of disease. All patients required transfusions. Seventy-six patients fulfilled all 4 criteria for severe aplastic anemia as proposed by Camitta [1]. Six patients had severe thrombocytopenia, a hypocellular bone marrow and borderline erythropoietic and granulopoietic function.

Group A: Bone marrow transplantation

Thirty-one patients had a matched sibling donor. Twenty-eight of them were primarily treated with bone marrow transplantation. Three patients were given immunosuppression due to unavailability or severe illness of the donor. In 2, bone marrow transplantation was performed later, after failure of antilymphocyte globulin therapy. It failed in both (Table 3). All patients given bone marrow transplantation were conditioned with cyclophosphamide, $4 \times 50\,mg/kg$. Twenty-one patients received unirradiated donor buffy coat after marrow transplantation. The first 14 patients were given methotrexate for prophylaxis of Graft-versus-Host-

Table 1. Classification criteria and treatment.

Group	Criteria	Initial criteria		
		Initial treatment		Changes in therapy
A	HLA–A, –B, –Dr identical sibling donor, mixed leukocyte culture not reactive	Cyclophosphamide (Cy) 50 mg/kg × 4 + bone marrow transplantation Methotrexate for GvHD prophylaxis		— add buffy coat (BC) — Cyclosporin (CyA) instead of Methotrexate (MTX)
B	HLA-haploidentical, ABO-identical, cross-match negative family donor	Antilymphocyte globulin (ALG) 40 mg/kg × 4 + bone marrow infusion (BMI) Norethandrolone (NA) 0.5–1 mg/kg/day by mouth		— add high dose Methylprednisolone (HdMP) — stop BMI
C	No donor	Antilymphocyte globulin (ALG) 40 mg/kg × 4 Norethandrolone (NA) 0.5–1 mg/kg/day by mouth		— add high dose Methylprednisolone (HdMP)

Group		Groups for analysis	
	principal therapy	subgroups	Therapy
A	Cy + BMT	A1	Cy + BMT, MTX
		A2	Cy + BMT + BC, MTX
		A3	Cy + BMT + BC, CyA
B	ALG + NA	B1	ALG + NA
		B2	ALG + NA + BMI
		B3	ALG + NA + BMI + HdMP
		B4	ALG + NA + HdMP

Disease [31], the subsequent 14 patients, starting in July 1979, were given cyclosporine [20–22].

Group B: Antilymphocyte globulin

Seventy-two patients were treated with antilymphocyte globulin. until July 1981, patients were given an infusion of bone marrow from a HLA-haplotype identical family donor after antilymphocyte globulin, if such a donor with negative cross-match was available. This bone marrow infusion was based on a beneficial effect seen in animal models after such an infusion [23–25]. During the study, it became apparent that this procedure did not improve survival in humans. In addition, the heparinized bone marrow may have been the cause of fatal intracerebral hemorrhage in two patients. The bone marrow infusion was therefore omitted from the protocol. The two groups (with and without mismatched bone marrow after antilymphocyte globulin) are therefore analyzed together. In 24 patients (group B3, B4, Table 1) high dose methylprednisolone was added in an attempt to enhance autologous recovery [25]. Methylprednisolone was given 1 g as a 24-hour-infusion from day 1 to 4, 0.5 g as a 24-hour-infusion from day 5 to 8, followed by oral prednisone 100 mg for 8 days, 75 mg for 8 days, followed by 5 mg daily for another 14 days. In all patients treated with antilymphocyte globulin since January 1976, oral norethandrolone (Nilevar R) 0, 5–1, 0 mg/kg daily was started on day 5 and maintained until signs of hemopoietic recovery occurred. Thereafter the dose was gradually reduced and kept on a maintenance dose of a minimum of 30 mg per week.

Equine antilymphocyte globulin from the same institute was used throughout the study. This antilymphocyte globulin (Lymphoser R) was manufactured by the Schweizerisches Serum- und Impfinstitut, Bern. It is produced by injecting horses with human thoracic duct lymphocytes. Initially we used serum from one horse, subsequently several batches consisting of pooled sera from at least three horses were used.

Supportive care

All patients treated with marrow transplantation were nursed in sterile laminar air flow units. Patients treated with antilymphocyte globulin stayed in single rooms with reverse isolation. Normally gastrointestinal decontamination was not attempted in these patients except for fungal prophylaxis. Patients left the hospital as soon as they were afebrile without antibiotics. They stayed in Basel as outpatients for daily examinations until self-sustaining hematopoiesis. The hemoglobin was kept above 8 g/dl and platelets above $20 \times 10/1$. Infections were treated immediately with appropriate antibiotics and, if required, with granulocyte transfusions.

Splenectomy Patients with prolonged thrombocytopenia and frequent need for platelet transfusions underwent splenectomy to facilitate support and decrease the need for platelet transfusions.

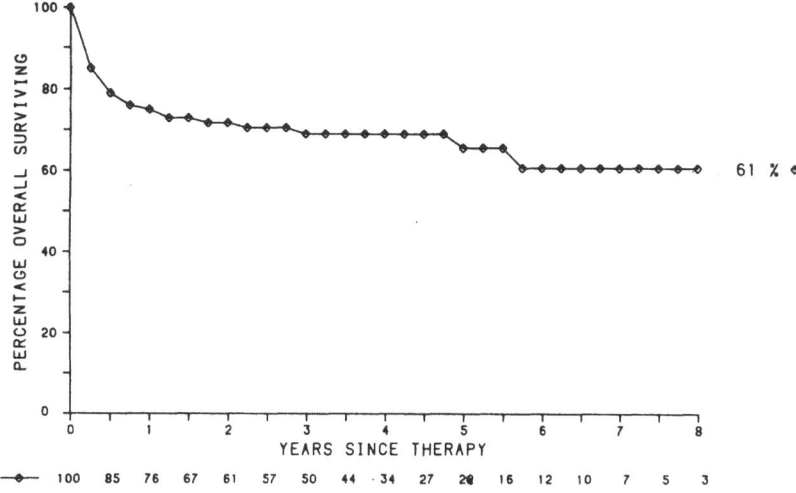

Figure 1. Survival according to Kaplan Meier of all 100 patients.

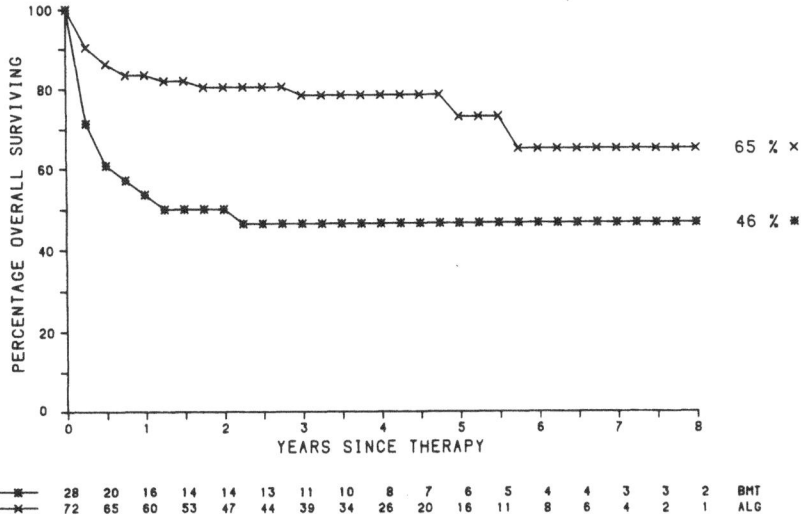

Figure 2. Comparison of patients treated with ALG (×) and patients treated with BMT (★). Survival according to Kaplan Meier.

Results

The overall probability of survival at 8 years for the total 100 patients is 61% (Figure 1). Survival curves for patients treated with bone marrow transplantation (= group A) and antilymphocyte globulin therapy (= group B) showed characteristic differences (Figure 2). After bone

Table 2. Hematological values of living patients (as of October 1, 1984).

Group	No. of patients	Hemoglobin (g/dl)	Granulocytes $\times 10^9/l$	Thrombocytes $\times 33^9/l$		Total
A	13	$\geqslant 12\,g\%$:13	$\geqslant 1,5 \times 10^9/l$:13	$\geqslant 100 \times 10^9/l$:13	CR	13
		$< 12\,g\%$:0	$< 1,5 \times 10^9/l$:0	$< 100 \times 10^9/l$:0	subnormal	0
B	53	$\geqslant 12\,g\%$:46	$\geqslant 1,5 \times 10^9/l$:36	$\geqslant 100 \times 10^9/l$:37	CR	36
		$< 12\,g\%$:7	$< 1,5 \times 10^9/l$:17	$< 100 \times 10^9/l$:16	subnormal	17

marrow transplantation, there was a 50% early treatment related complications. At two years, the survival curve reaches a stable plateau at 46%. There were no late fatal complications after bone marrow transplantation. Results of bone marrow transplantation for severe aplastic anemia improved with the introduction of cyclosporine for prevention of Graft-versus-Host-Disease. As shown in Figure 3, 5 of 14 patients given methotrexate are alive (36%), two of them with chronic Graft-versus-Host-Disease. Eight of 14 (57%) survive without chronic Graft-versus-Host-Disease with cyclosporine. All 13 surviving transplant patients have normal blood counts (Table 2).

The clinical course and causes of death are given in Table 3. Graft-versus-Host-Disease and cytomegalovirus infection remain the major causes of death in the transplant group. After antilymphocyte globulin therapy survival was 80% during the first 2 1/2 years. No apparent plateau was reached however, due to late complications such as paroxysmal nocturnal hemoglobinuria or relapse and the probability of survival at 8 years declines to 65% (Figure 2). As of October 1, 52 of 53 surviving patients from this group were self-sustaining and off transfusions but a

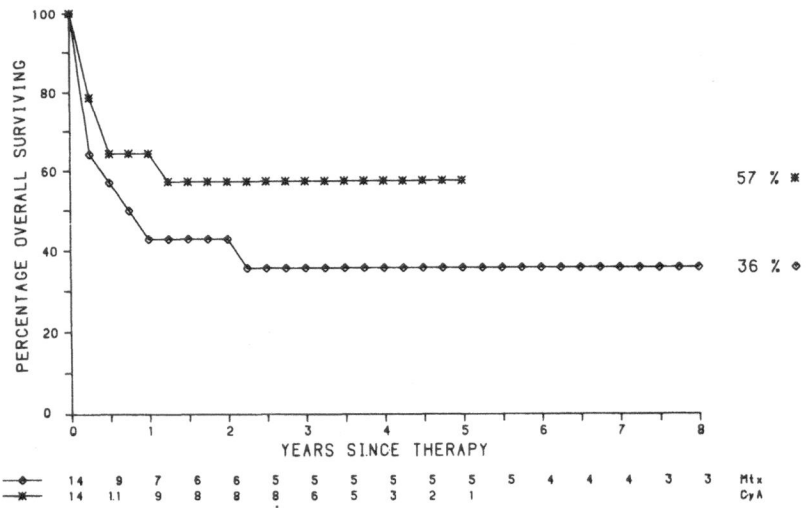

Figure 3. Comparison of BMT patients with prophylaxis against GvHD with MTX (⊠) or CyA (★). Survival according to Kaplan Meier.

Table 3. Results.

Group	No.	alive	Status	Dead	Cause of death
1	7	3	2 a/w chimeras, 1 a/w autologous recovery	4	2 infections, 1 rejection, 1 IP + GvHD
A 2	7	2	2 chronic GvHD, extensive disease	5	2 GvHD, 2 IP + GvHD, 1 infection
3	14	8	1 mild chronic GvHD, 7 a/w	6	1 CMV, 3 GvHD, 1 cardiac failure, 1 rejection
A	28	13 (46%)		15 (54%)	
1	17	11	10 a/w, 1 liver cell carcinoma	6	3 infections, 2 intracranialhemorrhages, 1 GvHD
2	31	21	1 PNH, 1 steroid dependent, 19 a/w	10	4 intracranialhemorrhages, 2 no response, 1 AML, 1 PNH, 1 infection, 1 relapse
B 3	5	5	1 steroid dependent, 1 PNH, 3 a/w	—	
4	19	16	1 PNH, 14 a/w, 1 platelet transfusions	3	1 infection, 1 intracranial hemorrage, 1 no response
B	72	53 (75%)		19 (25%)	
Total	100	66 (66%)		34 (34%)	

Table 4. Additional therapies.

Therapy because of no response after initial therapy

Initial therapy		No. of patients	Second therapy	Alive	Outcome
Group A	A 1	1	second BMT	—	IP + GvHD
		1	ALG	—	no response
	A 3	1	ALG + HdMP	—	no response
Group B	B 1	2	BMT	—	infection, GvHD
		1	ALG + BMI	1	a/w
		1	ALG	1	a/w
	B 4	4	ALG + HdMP	2	1 a/w, 1 needs platelet transfusions/2 died: 1 no response, 1 intracranial hemorrhage
Total		11		4	

Second therapy for relapse after initial response

Initial therapy		No. of patients	Second therapy	Alive	Outcome
Group A		0			
Group B	B 1	1	ALG + BMI	1	1 a/w (developed hepatocellular carcinoma, CR months after surgery and withdrawal of androgens)
		1	ALG + HdMP × 3	—	died after 4th course of ALG due to 3rd relapse
	B 2	4	ALG	1	1 a/w, 3 died: 1 PNH, 1 no response, 1 intracerebral hemorrhage
		3	ALG + HdMP	3	1: steroid dependent, 1 PNH, 1 required 3 courses of ALG + HdMP
	B 3	1	ALG + HdMP	1	steroid dependent
	B 4	1	ALG + HdMP	1	a/w (after 3rd ALG + HdMP)
Total		11		7	
Total		22		11	

fraction still had subnormal peripheral blood counts (Table 2). Twenty-two of the 100 original patients required additional therapy due to failure of either bone marrow transplantation or immunosuppression. As shown in Table 4, 3 patients from group A, were given either a second bone marrow transplant or antilymphocyte globulin. None of these patients survived.

In contrast, additional treatment after failture or initial antilymphocyte globulin resulted in a substantial number of responses. Eight patients who had not or only partially responded to a first course of antilymphocyte globulin were retreated (Table 4). Four are alive, 2 of them in complete autologous remission. In all 11 patients, severe aplastic anemia relapsed after initial response. Seven of them responded to a second course of antilymphocyte globulin and they are alive today. However, 3 with major complications (Table 4).

Splenectomy was performed in 26 patients to facilitate supportive care. No problems were associated with splenectomy. In 5 patients reduction of norethandrolone was followed by decrease of peripheral blood counts. Its dose was increased again in 4 patients and in a 5th patient prednisolone. was added. All 5 recovered hemopoietic function.

Discussion

The prognosis for patients with severe aplastic anemia has greatly improved during the last decade [1, 2, 4, 6, 8, 10, 14, 26, 28, 31]. From an almost invariably lethal outcome with supportive care alone or with androgens, treatment success has increased to the range of 80% at optimal conditions. Marrow transplantation performed early in untransfused young patients offers a long term cure rate between 70 and 80% [28, 29]. There are two major limitations to this optimistic outlook. The majority of patients does not have a HLA-identical sibling donor and very few patients are referred untransfused to transplant centers. In our study two of 28 patients only were not given transfusions before admission. Chronic Graft-versus-Host-Disease is also of concern. Two of our 5 patients given methotrexate are suffering from this problem while none of the 8 patients given cyclosporine is. These numbers are too small to draw any firm conclusions.

Treatment with antilymphocyte globulin with or without high dose steroids offers a true alternative to marrow transplantation. This approach, pioneered by Mathé [15] and confirmed by our own studies [13, 19, 26, 27] is now established in the treatment of severe aplastic anemia. A randomized study carried out at UCLA has demonstrated the value of antilymphocyte globulin therapy compared to treatment with supportive care alone. Eleven of 21 patients treated in this study with antilymphocyte globulin recovered. In contrast none of 21 patients given supportive care alone improved their counts during a three months observation period [5]. A cooperative randomized study demonstrated similar results: 76% of patients survived after treatment with antilymphocyte globulin compared to only 31% at 2 years in the control group [2]. A pilot study in Seattle as well as other open studies showed remission rates with antilymphocyte globulin therapy between 40 and 66% [7, 9, 12, 14, 18].

The results of our first 50 patients in 1981 [19] showed that treatment with antilymphocyte globulin was better or at least as effective as marrow transplantation in improving survival. This remains true in an extended number of patients. A few of the open questions have been clarified: the bone marrow infusion given initially in combination with antilymphocyte globulin (without the aim of engraftment) was based on experimental studies [23, 24, 25]. At the beginning of the study we had the impression that remissions were more complete if bone marrow infusion was added to antilymphocyte globulin, particularly since a few patients responded after initial failure of antilymphocyte globulin alone. Analysis of the results of a larger number of patients did not substantiate these initial assumptions, nor could others show a beneficial effect of the bone marrow infusion [7, 9]. We therefore discontinue the bone marrow infusion.

Thomas and Storb evaluated the advantages and disadvantages of antilymphocyte globulin therapy and bone marrow transplantation [30]. Our study confirms their conclusions. Antilymphocyte globulin can be given to any patient with severe aplastic anemia with a high chance of response. At two years, survival is significantly higher than after marrow transplantation. At five years the survival curve is still significantly better with the log rank test ($p < 0.025$) but not with the chi square test ($p > 0.1$). Patients treated with marrow transplantation usually recover normal hematopoiesis in vivo and in vitro and can be considered cured except those with chronic Graft-versus-Host-disease. Patients treated with antilymphocyte globulin in contrast, retain hematological abnormalities. Platelet and granulocyte counts are lower than normal, red cells show macrocytosis and bone marrow morphology continues to show stigmata of the disease: lymphocytic infiltrates and increased mast cells. Accordingly in vitro growth does not normalize [17]. Late disorders are of special concern: relapse and clonal hematological disorders such as paroxysmal nocturnal hemoglobinuria and leukemia can occur. They do, however, not reduce the value of antilymphocyte globulin therapy: survival and recovery from aplastic anemia can be induced and patients can lead a normal life for many years.

Open questions remain: initially androgens were given on the basis of anecdotal positive experience [1]. Although androgens per se clearly do not alter the course of severe aplastic anemia [3], they can be helpful in milder forms of aplastic and refractory anemias [16]. It is conceivable that they can have an effect in combination with antilymphocyte globulin therapy. We saw relapses after withdrawal or reduction of androgens and also a decrease of peripheral blood counts upon reduction of androgen dose. They increased after increase of the androgen dose. This explains why we keep all out-patients on low dose androgens, i.e. at a minimum of 10 mg three times a week. So far we were reluctant to withdraw this minimal dose completely, but recently one patient developed hepatoma with a likely relationship to androgen-therapy.

We conclude from our study that treatment with antilymphocyte globulin is a therapy with a good chance to survive with adequate bone marrow function and to lead a normal life. Results are better or at least equivalent to marrow transplant and patients with donors should be given the option of transplant or antilymphocyte globulin.

Acknowledgments

This investigation was supported by Grant No. 3.908.083 from the Swiss Science Foundation.

References

1. Camitta BM, Storb R, Thomas ED: Aplastic anemia. Pathogenesis, Diagnosis, Treatment and Prognosis. N Engl J Med 306:645–652, 712–718, 1982.
2. Camitta BM: A controlled prospective trial with antithoracic duct lymphocyte globulin (ATDLG) for treatment of severe aplastic anemia. Prog Clin Biol Res, 239–247, 1984.
3. Camitta BM, Thomas Ed, Nathan JG: A prospective study of androgens and bone marrow transplantation for treatment of severe aplastic anemia. Blood 53:504–514, 1979.
4. Champlin R, Ho W, Bayever E: Treatment of aplastic anemia: Results with bone marrow transplantation, antithymocyte globulin and monoclonal anti-T cell antibody. Prog Clin Biol Res 148:227–238, 1984.
5. Champlin R, Ho W, Gale RP: Antithymocyte globulin treatment in patients with aplastic anemia: A prospective randomized trial. N Engl J Med 308:113–118, 1983.
6. Doney KC, Torok-Storb B, Dahlberg S: Immunosuppressive therapy of severe aplastic anemia. Prog Clin Biol Res 148:259–270, 1984.
7. Doney KC, Weiden PL, Buckner CD: Treatment of severe aplastic anemia using antithymocyte globulin with or without an infusion of HLA haploidentical marrow. Exp Hematol 9:829–834, 1981.
8. Gluckman E, Devergie A, Berbunan A: Bone marrow transplantation in severe aplastic anemia using cyclophosphamide and thoracoabdominal irradiation. Prog Clin Biol Res 148:239–247, 1984.
9. Gluckman E, Devergie A, Poros A, Degoulet P: Results of immunosuppression in 170 cases of severe aplastic anemia: Report of the European Group of Bone marrow Transplant (EGBMT). Br J Haematol 51:541–550, 1982.
10. Gordon-Smith EC: Treatment of aplastic anemia. Prog Clin Biol Res 148:335–341, 1984.
11. Gratwhol A, Müller M, Osterwalder B, Burri HP, Nissen C, Jeannet M, Speck B: Treatment of severe aplastic anemia with combined antilymphocyte globulin and high dose methylprednisolone. Exp Hematol 10 (Suppl 11): 139:1982.
12. Jansen J, Zwaan FE, Haak HL: Antithymocyte globulin treatment for aplastic anemia. Scand J Haematol 28:341–351, 1982.
13. Jeannet M, Rubinstein AS, Pelet B, Kummer H: Prolonged remission of severe aplastic anemia after ALG pretreated and HLA-semi incompatible bone marrow cell transfusion. Transpl Proc 6:359–363, 1974.

14. Marmont Am, Bacigalupo A, van Lint MT: Treatment of severe aplastic anemia with high dose methylprednisolone and antilymphocyte globulin. Prog Clin Biol Res 148:271–287, 1984.
15. Mathé G, Amiel JL, Schwarzenberg L: Bone marrow grafts in man after conditioning by antilymphocyte serum. Br Med J i:131–136, 1970.
16. Najean Y: Long term follow up in patients with aplastic anemia. Amer J Med 71:543–551, 1981.
17. Nissen C, Cornu P, Gratwhol A, Speck B: Peripheral blood cells from patients with aplastic anemia in partial remission supress growth of their own bone marrow precursors in culture. Br J Haematol 45:233–243, 1980.
18. Rothmann SA, Streeter RR, Bukowski RM, Hewlett JS: Treatment of severe aplastic anemia with antithymocyte globulin. Exp Hematol 10:809–816, 1982.
19. Speck B, Gratwohl A, Nissen C: Treatment of severe aplastic anemia with antilymphocyte globulin or bone marrow transplantation. Br Med J 282:860–863, 1981.
20. Speck B, Gratwohl A, Nissen C: Cyclosporin-A for prophylaxis of GvHD in clinical bone marrow transplantation. Exp Hematol Today 3:117–120, 1981.
21. Speck B, Gratwohl A, Nissen C: Bone marrow grafting for leukaemia and aplastic anaemia. In DJG White (ed) Cyclosporin-A. Amsterdam, New York, Oxford: Elsevier Biomedical Press, 1981, pp 491–496.
22. Speck B, Gratwohl A, Nissen C: Knochenmarktransplantation bei Leukämie und aplastischer Anämie. Schweiz Med Wschr 113:622–629, 1983.
23. Speck B, Buckner CD, Cornu P, Jeannet M: Rationale for the use of ALG as sole immunosuppressant in allogeneic bone marrow transplantation for aplastic anemia. Transplant Proc 8:617–622, 1976.
24. Speck B, Kissling M: Successful bone marrow grafts in experimental aplastic anaemia using antilymphocyte serum for conditioning. Eur J Clin Biol Res 10:1047–1051, 1971.
25. Speck B, Cornu P, Nissen C: On the pathogenesis and treatment of aplastic anemia. Exp Hematol Today 2:143–149, 1978.
26. Speck B, Gratwohl A, Nissen C: Treatment of severe aplastic anemia: a prospective study of antilymphocyte globulin versus bone marrow transplantation. Prog Clin Biol Res 148:249–258, 1984.
27. Speck B, Gluckman E, Haak HL, van Rood JJ: Treatment of aplastic anaemia by antilymphocyte globulin with and without allogeneic bone marrow infusions. Lancet ii:1145–1148, 1977.
28. Storb R, Thomas ED, Appelbaum FR: Marrow transplantation for severe aplastic anemia: The Seattle experience. Prog Clin Biol Res 148:297–313, 1984.
29. Storb R, Thomas ED, Buckner CD: Marrow transplantation in 30 "untransfused" patients with severe aplastic anemia. Ann Intern Med 92:30–36, 1980.
30. Thomas ED, Storb R: Perspective: Acquired severe aplastic anaemia: Progress and perplexity. Blood 64:325–328, 1984.
31. Thomas ED, Storb R, Clift RA, Fefer A, Johnson FL, Neiman PE, Lerner KG, Glucksberg H, Buckner CD: Bone marrow transplantation. N Engl J Med 292:832–843, 895–902, 1975.
32. Young N, Speck B: Antithymocyte and antilymphocyte globulines: Clinical trials and mechanism of action. Prog Clin Biol Res 148:221–226, 1984.